STARTLI...

- 1 in 2 men and 1 in 3 women will develop cancer in their lifetimes
- Over one million new cases of cancer are diagnosed each year
- Since 1990, there have been 11 million new cancer cases diagnosed—five million of those resulted in death
- This year, over half a million Americans will die of cancer—more than 1500 people a day
- After heart disease, cancer is the leading cause of death in the U.S.
- One in four U.S. deaths is from cancer
- **One-third of cancer deaths in this country are nutrition-related**

DON'T BE A STATISTIC—FIGHT CANCER WITH . . .

THE BROCCOLI SPROUTS BREAKTHROUGH

THE
BROCCOLI SPROUTS BREAKTHROUGH

THE NEW MIRACLE FOOD FOR CANCER PREVENTION

DEBORAH MITCHELL

A LYNN SONBERG BOOK

St. Martin's Paperbacks

THE BROCCOLI SPROUTS BREAKTHROUGH

Copyright © 1998 by Lynn Sonberg Book Associates.

ISBN: 0-312-96846-9

Printed in the United States of America

St. Martin's Paperbacks edition / October 1998

St. Martin's Paperbacks are published by St. Martin's Press, 175 Fifth Avenue, New York, NY 10010.

10 9 8 7 6 5 4 3 2 1

A Note to Readers

This book is for informational purposes only. Readers are advised to consult a trained medical professional before acting on any of the medical information in this book. The fact that an organization is listed in Appendix A to the book does not mean that the author or publisher recommends the organization or endorses any of the services or advice it may offer or suggest.

Contents

1. Broccoli Sprouts—Nature's Weapon Against Cancer

THEY STAND ABOUT TWO TO THREE INCHES TALL, ARE FRAIL and spindly, fall over in the slightest breeze . . . and are a powerful force against the second leading cause of death in the United States—cancer. They are broccoli sprouts, the newest natural weapon for cancer prevention. These incredible greens are waiting for you on an increasing number of grocery store shelves right now. With the help of this book, you can easily make them a healthful addition to your life.

Cancer is an equal opportunity disease: It strikes people of all ages, races, economic means, and religions and can affect any part of the body. But you have the ability to reduce your chances of getting cancer if you follow some easy guidelines. One precaution you can adopt is eating healthful, organic food. Approximately one-third of cancer deaths are related to the food we eat. But take heart! Although some foods are known to be harmful to your health, many more actually promote it. Scientists have identified many foods that have disease-fighting and health-protecting abilities. Broccoli sprouts are the newest addition to this category of foods—and they are causing quite a stir. That's because eating as little as one-quarter ounce of broccoli sprouts daily could reduce your chances of getting cancer by 20, 30, or even as much as 50 percent. And for anyone who doesn't like broccoli, there's even more good news: The sprouts don't taste like their grown-up version!

HOW TO TAKE ADVANTAGE OF THE BROCCOLI SPROUTS BREAKTHROUGH

This book is a comprehensive overview of the broccoli sprout breakthrough in cancer prevention. You will learn exciting information about how scientists discovered the "magic" contained in these tiny greens, and how they prevent cancer. Tips on how you can grow your own sprouts at home and purchase the safest, most nutritious sprouts and other disease- and cancer-fighting foods on the market are also covered. The "main course" of the book shows you how you can incorporate broccoli sprouts into your diet so you can enjoy them and reap their benefits. And because no one can live by sprouts alone—no matter how good they taste— this course includes information about many other health-promoting foods as well. In Chapter 7 you get a full two weeks' worth of menus and recipes that use broccoli sprouts and the many other delicious foods discussed in this book. The book concludes with several chapters dedicated to helping you choose the healthiest sprouts and other disease-fighting foods, and a detailed discussion on how you can take control of your health and reduce your risk of cancer and other diseases.

First, let's take a brief introductory look at the two areas that are the focus of this book: the world of sprouts and the often deadly disease they can help prevent—cancer.

SPROUT POWER

Sprouts are the newborns of the plant world: the fragile yet hardy tendrils that emerge from a seed. Although most plants progress beyond the sprouting stage and grow into mature adults, some are plucked or harvested as sprouts for food. Mung bean sprouts, a popular ingredient in Oriental food, and alfalfa sprouts, a common sandwich topping, are just two types often seen on produce shelves. Some people cultivate the sprouts of lentils, soybeans, wheat, peas, radishes, and various other grains, legumes, and vegetables and make them a part of their daily fare. That's because these sprouts are powerhouses of nutrients, like taking a "green" vitamin and mineral supplement. They are an excellent addition to any diet, and later in this book you will learn how to make them a part of yours.

The introduction of broccoli to the sprout scene has caused a lot of fanfare because these new vegetables offer a bright ray of hope. Nutritionists, scientists, and others in the medical field have known for many years that eating fruits and vegetables can help reduce the risk of cancer and other diseases (more on this in Chapter 3). But many people don't eat the recommended five or more servings per day of these healthful foods (see Chapter 4). Wouldn't it be great if you could get the benefits of much of those servings in a handful of sprouts? Just one ounce of broccoli sprouts contains the same amount of a potent cancer-fighting substance, called sulforaphane, as two pounds of broccoli. When made a part of a healthful diet and lifestyle, broccoli sprouts may be the most powerful cancer-fighter you can eat. For example, studies show that you can reduce your risk of colon cancer by 50 percent by eating two pounds of broccoli and similar vegetables a week. Now you can get the same amount of protection from about one ounce of broccoli sprouts per week: toss a few sprouts on your sandwich or salad or stir a few into your soup each day.

CANCER: UP CLOSE AND PERSONAL

It's rare to find someone who has not been touched in some way by cancer. You may have a family member, friend, coworker, or neighbor with the disease, or you may have cancer yourself. If you are a woman, the probability that you will develop cancer during your lifetime is one in three; if you're a man, the risk is higher: one in two. These alarming risk rates have not always been so high. In 1900, 4 percent of all deaths in the United States were attributed to cancer. By 1970, that figure was 17 percent, and only twenty years later it rose to 24 percent. What will that percentage be in another 20 years?

We all have a voice and a stake in whether that percentage goes down or continues to rise. Fortunately, everyone can significantly reduce his or her own risk of developing cancer. For some people the effort can be as easy as making a few dietary changes; for others, it may involve quitting smoking, reducing exposure to the sun, or changing jobs to get away from a toxic environment (see Chapter 8). But everyone can start with a simple, convenient, tasty, and important step: adding broccoli sprouts to their daily "to do" list to help fight cancer. One look at cancer statistics reveals how challenging an opponent it is.

CANCER: A GROWING PROBLEM

- Approximately 1.4 million new cases of cancer occur each year in the United States.

- Cancer is the second leading cause of death in the United States; heart disease is the first.

- In 1996, approximately 10 million cases of cancer occurred around the world. That number is expected to reach 14.7 million within the next twenty years.

- More than 1,500 Americans die of cancer each day.

- Lung cancer affects one in twelve men and one in eighteen women.

- Colon and rectal cancer affect one in seventeen men and women.

- One in eight women can expect to develop breast cancer.

- One in five men can expect to develop prostate cancer.

- More than 900,000 cases of skin cancer are diagnosed every year.
- High-protein diets (typically from high meat consumption), especially when combined with high-fat foods, are associated with an increased risk of cancer of the breast, prostate, colon, pancreas, kidney, and uterus.
- Smokers are ten times more likely to develop lung cancer than nonsmokers.

THE LINK BETWEEN CANCER AND DIET

Thousands of research studies have been conducted over the past several decades on the effects of diet on cancer risk, prevention, and prognosis. The Diet & Cancer Project, an ambitious four-year collaborative effort between the American Institute for Cancer Research and the World Cancer Research Fund, has brought this wealth of data together. The fifteen leading experts in diet and cancer who conducted this massive project reviewed more than 4,500 research studies and consulted with more than 120 health professionals from around the world.

The 660-page report issued by the project, "Food, Nutrition and the Prevention of Cancer: A Global Perspective," is the first ever to focus on whole diets and food, not just specific elements within foods, and the first to analyze the connection between food and cancer prevention from a worldwide view. According to the American Institute for Cancer Research, this report "will help set new directions in research, cancer education and public health policy for years to come, both in the U.S. and around the world." The report examines the relationship between what we eat and drink and eighteen common types of cancer. It also provides specific dietary recommendations for cancer prevention, which I discuss in detail in Chapter 4.

For now, the most important message to take from this landmark project is this: **Cancer is preventable.** Thirty to

40 percent of all cancers are directly linked to the food we eat, the amount of exercise we get, and how we maintain our weight. These figures are in alignment with those of the National Cancer Institute, which estimates that 35 percent of all cancer deaths are associated with diet.

Knowing that food plays such a primary role in cancer, it is important that the food you and your family eat is not only healthy and nutritious but also helps fight cancer and other disease. Making cancer-fighting foods a regular part of your diet is not an iron-clad guarantee that you or your loved ones will never get cancer, but with the solid scientific knowledge that simple changes in dietary choices can result in a reduction in death, suffering, and medical expenses, the path to better health seems clear.

A BRIEF HISTORY OF BROCCOLI SPROUTS

More than twenty years ago, scientists discovered that certain vegetables have the power to prevent cancer. This was a significant finding, because it indicated that people could reduce their risk of cancer by eating, or not eating, certain foods. At the time, those conducting the research had not identified what was responsible for this benefit.

Then in 1992, a team of researchers at Johns Hopkins Medical Institute, led by Paul Talalay, M.D., said they had found a possible explanation for the anticancer power. Vegetables in the Brassica family, which are often referred to as cruciferous vegetables and include broccoli and cauliflower, contain sulforaphane, a chemical that stimulates the body's natural ability to fight cancer. Of all the cruciferous plants, which also include arugula, bok choy, brussels sprouts, cabbage, Chinese cabbage, collards, cress, daikon, kale, kohlrabi, mustard, turnip, and watercress, the plant with the highest concentration of sulforaphane is broccoli.

Armed with this information, the researchers decided to go farther: They wanted to increase the level of sulforaphane in broccoli. They soon found, however, that among the approximately eighty varieties of broccoli, the amount of sulforaphane varies greatly. In fact, only one-third of broccoli varieties contain a high level of sulforaphane. Then as the scientists worked diligently in the laboratory to grow a "better" strain of broccoli, they made an unexpected discovery: The fragile three-day-old broccoli sprouts contained up to one hundred times the level of sulforaphane found in mature broccoli. On average per unit weight, broccoli sprouts have twenty- to fifty-fold greater anticancer activity than does mature broccoli. Scientists didn't have to improve on Nature; she had had the answer all along.

To test the potency of the sprouts, Talalay and his team studied two groups of rats. One group received extracts of broccoli sprouts for five days; the other group—the controls—did not. Both groups were then exposed to a carcinogen called dimethylbenzanthracene. About 40 percent of the controls developed breast tumors within 100 days of exposure to the carcinogen, compared with only 20 percent of the treated rats. Of the treated rats that did develop tumors, the growths were fewer in number, smaller, and took longer to develop. The scientists knew they had made an important discovery.

BRINGING THE SPROUTS FROM THE LAB TO YOU

The exciting findings of the animal study led Dr. Talalay to speculate that broccoli sprouts could fight cancer in people as well. Now the task was to bring the sprouts to market. That's when Dr. Talalay's team did something that is rare in the health food market: they created a nonprofit organization, the Brassica Foundation for Cancer Protection Research, which will donate all profits from selling the sprouts to cancer research. The foundation will also work with commercial growers to test their sprouts to ensure they are of the highest potency and quality. This step is necessary because the potency of sulforaphane varies greatly among broccoli varieties.

While Dr. Talalay continues to test broccoli sprouts in

his laboratories, commercial growers are eager to get their product to market. One of the largest entries is the Brassica Sprout Group, a joint venture between Brassica Protection Products and the Sholl Group, which licenses the Green Giant name. Brassica Protection Products has its own laboratory staff who rigorously test and certify the level of sulforaphane in the sprouts they grow. According to Jeff Sholl, president of the Sholl Group, the broccoli sprouts released under the Green Giant name "are grown under rigorous certification procedures," which will ensure that the sprouts "contain scientifically established levels of sulforaphane."

Broccoli sprouts have begun to "crop up" on supermarket shelves around the country. If you don't see them in your grocery store, check out natural food stores or health food stores. Or you can grow your own (see Chapter 6).

YOU AND BROCCOLI SPROUTS

That's the nutshell version of how broccoli sprouts broke into the health scene. But there is much more exciting information to share. The next chapter explores why many people are calling these sprouts the new miracle food for cancer prevention. You are invited to look at your eating habits and learn how you can incorporate broccoli sprouts and other health-promoting, cancer-fighting foods into your daily menus. You won't have to do this alone: Chapters 4 and 7 give you the latest information on "medicine" foods and how they can help prevent a wide range of diseases and keep you looking and feeling younger longer. Forget that old saying, "If it's good for you, it must not taste good." Although I can't guarantee that you'll love every recipe provided in this book, I think you'll come very close.

Broccoli sprouts are on the leading edge of natural health-promoting remedies. Simple yet powerful, they dare to challenge many of the high-tech approaches to cancer- and other disease-fighting methods. Yet at the same time, scientists are using the latest in testing, monitoring, and reporting technology to study, grow, and develop broccoli sprouts in order to deliver a truly valuable product to the general public. This effort is an example of how nature and technology can work together to bring you better health and longer life.

2. The Preventive Powers of Broccoli Sprouts

FOR MILLENNIA, PEOPLE HAVE KNOWN THAT CERTAIN FOODS have healing powers. But it has been only within the past few decades that scientists and researchers from the fields of nutrition and medicine have taken a serious, scientific look at not only *which* foods can prevent, treat, and cure disease but also *how* and *why* they can. Before these questions can be answered, it's important to appreciate what you are fighting. This chapter looks at the many facets of cancer and cancer research and the preventive powers of sulforaphane. It also offers a clear understanding of how including cancer- and disease-fighting foods in your diet can be one of the most wonderful gifts you can give yourself and your family: a gift of health and vitality and the feeling that you are in control of your well-being.

UNDERSTANDING CANCER

At one time, scientists and medical professionals thought of cancer as one disease entity. This perception influenced the way they approached treatment strategies. Now we know that *cancer* is an umbrella term for more than one hundred diseases that share a common characteristic: abnormal cell growth that gets out of control. Cancer can affect people of all ages, but it occurs most often in people older than fifty.

If the uncontrolled growth and spread of abnormal cells is not stopped, it can cause death.

Cancer does not appear overnight. According to Gary Stoner, professor of preventive medicine at Ohio State's Comprehensive Cancer Center, "Cancer is the accumulation of genetic alterations. It requires constant exposure to carcinogens. . . . Then it can take more than a decade for those mutated cells to become cancer cells." Thus it takes time for cancer to form, which means you have time to prevent it. And that time is now.

The Vocabulary of Cancer

Cancer is a complex topic, and it is easy to become confused by all the terms physicians use when talking about it. To help you better understand cancer and how it works, here is a miniature glossary of cancer-related terms:

Adenocarcinoma: carcinoma derived from glandular cells

Benign: noncancerous

Cancer staging: an identification system that describes how far cancer has spread throughout the body. There are two types of staging systems. One uses roman numerals I through IV: Stage I cancers are usually curable, while stage IV usually denotes inoperable disease. The TNM system (Tumor, Nodes, and Metastases) classifies the extent of each of these elements in any given case of cancer.

Carcinogen: something that causes cancer

Carcinogenesis: the transformation of normal cells into cancer cells

Carcinoma: cancer that develops in skin cells or in the cells in the lining (epithelial) of the lungs, organs, and mouth

Carcinoma in situ: very early stage tumor that is confined to a microscopic site. The body's immune system may or may not eventually destroy the cells.

Chemoprotection: intentionally fortifying the body's defense system against the effects of carcinogens

Dysplasia: describes abnormal cells that could, if untreated, become cancerous

Hodgkin's disease: a type of cancer in which the lymph nodes, spleen, liver, and often other body tissues become enlarged

Leukemia: cancer of the blood, bone marrow, and spleen

Lymphoma: cancer in the lymphatic system

Malignant: cancerous

Melanoma: a pigmented mole or tumor that may be benign or malignant

Metastasis: the movement of cancer cells from one part of the body to another

Multiple myeloma: a type of cancer in which tumors infiltrate the bone and bone marrow

Neoplasm: an abnormal growth, such as a tumor

Sarcoma: cancer of the connective tissue, cartilage, bone, and muscle that often affects the liver, kidneys, spleen, bladder, lungs, and parotids (salivary glands)

How Cancer Starts

During the normal life cycle of cells, old ones die and new ones take their place through a process of normal cell reproduction. This replacement process is predetermined by the genetic code found in the DNA of every cell. When all goes according to plan, the replacement cells are carbon copies of the dead cells, matching their shape, size, function, and number.

Sometimes, however, something goes wrong and the cells divide uncontrollably. (The "wrong" can be any number of factors, many of which are discussed in depth in Chapter 8.) Eventually these renegade cells form a tumor, known as the *primary tumor*. If cells break away from this primary tumor, they go elsewhere in the body and form *secondary tumors*. The location of the primary tumor determines the type of cancer. For example, a primary tumor in the liver that spreads cells to the breast is not breast cancer but "metastatic liver cancer"; the cancer cells have moved from one part of the body to another.

Just as there are many different types of cancer, there are

also many different causes of cancer. These causes fall into two main categories: external (radiation, processed foods, pesticides, alcohol, excess dietary fat, tobacco) and internal (hormones, inherited mutations). Any one or more of these and other factors can trigger uncontrolled cell growth. Because the topic of cancer risks—and how to avoid them or reduce their impact—is so important, it is discussed at length in Chapter 8.

Any given case of cancer is probably caused by more than one factor. That is why it is crucial for you to take a holistic approach to your health and consider adding broccoli sprouts and other cancer-fighting foods to your diet, along with routine exercise, stress management, weight control, and not smoking.

TREATMENT

The concept that cancer is really many diseases, rather than different types of the same disease, affecting each organ or site in a different way, has changed the way researchers seek treatments and cures, as well as the way physicians prescribe therapies. Such thinking has opened the doors to many different conventional as well as natural/holistic methods to deal with this body of diseases. Conventional medical treatments include radiation, chemotherapy (the use of drug therapy), and surgery. Often, radiation and chemotherapy are done on an outpatient basis, which allows patients to maintain a relatively normal lifestyle. Ill effects from such treatments, such as nausea, hair loss, and fatigue, are common but usually manageable.

Surgery to remove tumors and surrounding tissue is another option. An alternative type of surgery, called cryosurgery (or cryotherapy) is the use of extreme cold in the form of liquid nitrogen to destroy cancer cells. Traditionally it has been used to treat skin cancer, but recently physicians are evaluating its use in prostate and liver cancers and for some tumors of the brain, bone, and windpipe.

The use of natural cancer remedies and methods ·has

become more common in recent years. Those who practice alternative medicine believe that the underlying cause of cancers is an ineffective immune system. Therefore, the alternative methods used (which may include herbal medicine, nutritional support, meditation, and prayer) attempt to return the patient's immune system to a healthy functioning level. Because diet plays such a crucial role in the development of cancer, eating cancer-fighting foods, including the potent broccoli sprouts, is one of the most important things you can do.

Types of Cancer and Prevalence Rates

Tumors can appear anywhere in the body. The most common types of cancer and their prevalence rates are given in the box below.

TYPES OF CANCER AND PREVALENCE RATES*

Type	New Cases
Skin	900,000
Prostate	209,900
Breast	181,600
Lung	178,100
Colorectal	131,200 (94,100 are colon)
Bladder	54,500
Non-Hodgkin's lymphoma	53,600
Uterine (endometrium)	34,900
Oral and pharynx	30,750
Kidney	28,800
Leukemia	28,300
Pancreas	27,600
Ovary	26,800
Stomach	22,400
Brain	17,600

Thyroid	16,100
Cervix	14,500
Multiple myeloma	13,800
Liver	13,600
Esophagus	12,500
Larynx	10,900
Hodgkin's disease	7,500

*Source: National Council for Cancer Research, from Web site http://www.nfcr.org/cancerchart.html

A BRIEF HISTORY OF CANCER RESEARCH

Although cancer has existed for thousands of years, it was not accurately diagnosed until the early 1800s. Research into finding a cure began immediately. Formalized research has been going on for more than 140 years, and today there are many organizations and institutes conducting such work. Among them are the Institute of Cancer Research, established in 1909; the U.S. National Cancer Institute; the International Agency on Research in Cancer; the National Foundation for Cancer Research (1973); the Strang Cancer Prevention Center (1933); and the American Institute for Cancer Research (1982), which is responsible for the landmark Diet & Cancer Project discussed earlier. Each of these cancer organizations has a specific focus, and each can be credited with landmark "firsts" in cancer research, or significant contributions to the research effort (see box).

SOME CANCER RESEARCH "FIRSTS" AND ACCOMPLISHMENTS

- Strang Cancer Prevention Center: The Kate Depew Strang Clinic was the first clinic established for the early detection of cancer, the first medical facility to use the Pap test for early detection of cervical cancer, and the first to use sigmoidoscopy for the early detection of colon cancer.

- National Foundation for Cancer Research: Seven NFCR-supported researchers have received the Nobel Prize.

- Institute of Cancer Research: Made the first pure chemical carcinogens; carried out some of the first experimental research on carcinogenic oils and tars.

- American Institute for Cancer Research: "Author" of the Diet & Cancer Project; the only major national cancer charity that focuses exclusively on diet, nutrition, and cancer.

- National Cancer Institute: Along with the National Surgical Adjuvant Breast and Bowel Project, announced the first prevention trial in the world to show that a drug can reduce the incidence of breast cancer.

In the United States, a major effort to conquer cancer was initiated on December 23, 1971, when President Richard Nixon launched the "War on Cancer." When Nixon signed the National Cancer Act of 1971 into law, one of the results was the creation of the National Cancer Program. This program, coordinated by the National Cancer Institute, conducts and supports research, training, dissemination of information, and other programs concerned with the cause, diagnosis, prevention, and treatment of cancer; cancer rehabilitation; and continuing care of cancer patients and their families. Nixon believed that this effort and those of the many other cancer research institutions would result in a cure for cancer in about eight years.

Yet despite more than a quarter century of tireless research, the impact on the most common types of cancer— breast, prostate, colon, and lung—has been minimal. The overall cancer rate has risen: It was 18 percent higher in 1994 than it was in 1971. One reason this has happened, says Dr. Talalay, is that researchers and physicians failed to realize that even when a malignancy is first detected, the DNA has most likely been conducting its damage for many years, undetected in the body. The real work, he believes, is to stop or reverse the cell-damaging process. The key is control, protection, and prevention, and these are steps everyone can take, every day.

Every person, after all, is his or her own worst enemy. Anthony B. Miller of Toronto, Canada, an expert on preventive medicine, says, "We probably know enough already to prevent more than half of all cancers, if only we put our knowledge into effect."

The exciting and promising news is that the shift in research and the war on cancer is happening now. Whereas most research used to focus on finding a cure or better treatments, Dr. Talalay explains that the emphasis now is "to 'cure' cancer before it becomes a clinical problem." For about twenty years, Dr. Talalay and his colleagues have been doing just that. One major result of their work is the broccoli sprouts breakthrough.

Another sign of encouragement is that even though more people are getting cancer, they are living longer. In the early 1970s, 40 percent of people with cancer could expect to live at least five years; that percentage is now 50 percent. Early detection, possible because of the widespread use of tests such as mammograms and the Pap test for identifying cancer of the uterus and cervix, has helped bring the death rate from these cancers down 70 percent. Death from stomach cancer has been reduced by two-thirds since the Cancer Act was signed. New drugs may also hold some hope. Recently, researchers at the Children's Hospital in Boston found that two new drugs, angiostatin and endostatin, shrink tumors in mice by preventing the growth of new blood vessels to the tumors, thus starving them. Yet the key to the war on cancer remains control.

CONTROLLING CANCER: PREVENTION AND CHEMOPROTECTION

To control cancer, cancer experts recommend a twofold approach: prevention and chemoprotection. *Prevention* involves reducing or eliminating your exposure to cancer-causing (carcinogenic) substances. These include tobacco, pesticides and herbicides, alcohol, excessive dietary fat, radiation, and hundreds of industrial and other environmental toxins. *Chemoprotection* is the use of specific substances in a deliberate effort to boost the body's natural defense mechanisms and therefore reduce its susceptibility to cancer-causing agents. For the most effective control of cancer, you need to practice both of these empowering strategies. This book provides you with the needed tools. When you take advantage of these tools, you take control of your health and your future.

DIGGING DEEP FOR DISEASE-PREVENTIVE SUBSTANCES

Scientists know that, on a molecular level, one way to protect against cancer and other medical conditions in which the cells undergo some abnormal growth or mutation is to induce, or stimulate, the function of substances called phase II enzymes. Researchers in several laboratories are identifying and studying various "inducers," natural and laboratory-made, in an attempt to find the most potent cancer-fighting substances. The one of particular interest here is sulforaphane, a substance that belongs to a group of chemoprotectors known as phytochemicals, substances that protect plants from the damaging effects of too much sun. (This and other phytochemicals are currently under investigation for their cancer-blocking and other healing benefits; see Chapter 3.)

Sulforaphane is a specific type of phytochemical known as an isothiocyanate, which has the ability to promote the activity of phase II enzymes. For several years, nutrition experts and scientists have sung the praises of broccoli for its cancer-preventive powers, both before and after President George Bush admitted that he hated the green vegetable. Imagine the excitement, then, when Dr. Talalay and his team discovered that compared with mature broccoli, the three-day-old sprouts contain ten to one hundred times higher levels of the glucosinolate of sulforaphane. Glucosinolate is a precursor— a substance that comes before another substance and usually helps it develop or form, sort of like a mentor. The combination of glucosinolate and naturally occurring sulforaphane together give broccoli sprouts their superior cancer-fighting ability. As a bonus, not only don't the sprouts taste like broccoli, they also don't cause the gastrointestinal "feedback" many people experience with broccoli!

Talalay's team did give mature broccoli a good chance to prove itself. They ran tests on twenty-nine samples of fresh and frozen broccoli for the level of inducer activity in each. They chose both national and generic frozen brands as well as conventionally and organically grown fresh broccoli. Although levels of sulforaphane were higher in the fresh samples, the levels in sprouts were still far superior. This does not mean that mature broccoli is not a nutritious addition to any diet, especially if you love broccoli, but ounce for ounce, the sprouts definitely pack the cancer-fighting power.

But the investigators still had questions. Why are sulforaphane levels so high in sprouts and so much lower in the mature plant? How do the sulforaphane levels of other cruciferous plants compare with those of broccoli? How effective is the sulforaphane in broccoli sprouts in arresting cancer?

What the Investigators Found

Although researchers are not certain why sulforaphane is so concentrated in sprouts and then dramatically declines in mature plants, one theory is that the chemicals are needed to protect only very young plants. Once the plants mature, they can protect themselves, and so most of the sulforaphane disappears.

To determine the level of sulforaphane in other cruciferous plants, the scientists evaluated arugula, brussels sprouts, cabbage, cauliflower, Chinese cabbage, collards, daikon, kale, kohlrabi, mustard, red radish, turnip, and watercress. Broccoli consistently came up the winner with the highest level of inducer activity, making it the top candidate for further study. Cauliflower did make an impressive showing, however, so it's possible cauliflower sprouts could be sharing produce shelf space with their cousin in the near future.

To answer questions about sulforaphane's cancer-blocking properties, broccoli sprouts were put to the test in 1994 by Dr. Talalay and his team. As reported in Chapter 1, the rats that received sulforaphane fared much better than their untreated friends. Overall, rats given sulforaphane were 60 percent less likely to develop breast cancer, and the tumors that did appear in the treated rats were 75 percent smaller than those among untreated rats. Apparently, sulforaphane triggers production of phase II enzymes as the scientists had hoped. Phase II enzymes neutralize harmful chemicals that destroy DNA and make cells vulnerable to tumor growth.

At this point, sulforaphane's abilities seem to be confined to preventing cancer, rather than tackling it once it has developed. That means that broccoli sprouts have preventive rather than curative powers against cancer, making them an excellent choice in your personal war against this disease.

Talalay's findings so impressed the National Cancer Institute that the organization and several philanthropists supported the creation of the Brassica Chemoprotection Laboratory. The laboratory, headed by Dr. Talalay, has equipment able to test the chemoprotective properties of a wide variety of vegetables, fruits, and herbs. The laboratory is also equipped to select, breed, and cultivate plants with high chemoprotective abilities. In special indoor "gardens" with fluorescent lights, researchers in one week raise sprouts that have as much sulforaphane as one acre of broccoli would yield in one season.

Other Advantages of Broccoli Sprouts

Broccoli sprouts have another significant feature that makes them important in the fight against cancer. The "good guy" phase II enzymes have "bad guy" cousins, phase I enzymes, which have the potential to stimulate the growth of tumors. Compared with mature broccoli, the sprouts contain a minuscule amount of another precursor called indole glucosinolates, which induce phase I enzymes. But don't worry; the level of indole glucosinolates in mature broccoli is far outweighed by the amount of cancer-protectant sulforaphane it contains. The near lack of indole glucosinolates in the sprouts, however, strengthens the tiny greens' disease-fighting abilities.

Another plus associated with broccoli sprouts is that unlike the so-called designer foods and nutraceuticals now under development or on the market, broccoli sprouts are not genetically manipulated or enhanced: They are simply nature at its very (young) best.

The potent disease-fighting sulforaphane helps make broccoli sprouts a key element in cancer prevention. Yet these sprouts, along with dozens of other foods, contain other healing substances that can help you maintain your health. The next chapter takes a close look at some of these healing ingredients and the foods in which they are found.

3. Medicines in Your Meals: Foods That Fight Cancer and a Whole Lot More

SOME FOODS GIVE A WHOLE NEW MEANING TO THE TERM "FOOD fight." These are foods that fight *for* you when you consume them, because they contain substances that help safeguard you against disease. Included in this category are phytochemicals, antioxidants, fiber, and vitamins and minerals. Collectively, these disease-preventing components are often called nutraceuticals (from "nutrient" and "pharmaceutical"), a word whose first use has been credited to Stephen de Felice, M.D., director of New York's Foundation for Innovation in Medicine. Broccoli sprouts are a prime example of a food that provides nutraceuticals from all four categories, which makes it one of the best cancer- and disease-fighting foods you can eat.

As researchers learn more and more about the hundreds of nutraceuticals in food, it sometimes becomes difficult definitively to assign a substance to one class or another. Sometimes a nutrient conveniently fits into several categories; for example, beta-carotene is a phytochemical that acts as an antioxidant, and vitamin C is a vitamin that functions as an antioxidant.

Also, each major classification can have dozens of subclasses and sub-subclasses with hard-to-pronounce names. Rather than burden you with lots of terms, this chapter presents a basic structure that includes just enough identifying names to help you navigate through the maze of "medicine" foods and concentrates on how each of the health-promoting agents in those foods can work to protect you. (If you want more information about any of the substances discussed in this chapter, see Appendix B.) An overview of recommended daily requirements, and how much of each nutrient is suggested for optimal health, is presented in Chapter 4.

EAT TO YOUR HEALTH

How many fruits and vegetables did you eat today? How about yesterday? If you are like most Americans, you consumed fewer than the five or more servings recommended by the National Cancer Institute. Five or more servings is the *minimum* amount needed to reduce your risk of developing cancer by about 50 percent.

Fruits and vegetables supply an abundance of nutrients and fiber that are essential for preventing cancer and other diseases. To get the most benefit from these foods, choose a variety, including broccoli sprouts. Gladys Block, professor of public health at the University of California at Berkeley says, "There are some cancers for which one nutrient is more important than another. But then the opposite is true for another cancer. Nature packaged them all together in fruits and vegetables." The sections that follow describe some of the most important of Nature's nutritional gifts.

ANTIOXIDANTS

Antioxidant has become a household word over the last few years, and that's good, especially if you are including a sufficient amount of these nutrients in your daily diet. As often happens when a new health-related product hits the market, there is an information glut that leaves you with more questions than answers. The latest information about antioxidants presented below can help you answer those questions.

Antioxidants are any vitamins, minerals, or other nutrients that fight and disarm the harmful effects of damaging atoms in the body called free radicals. Although free radicals play a critical role in the metabolism and synthesis of carbohydrates, fat, and protein, they also can cause a great deal of damage in the body. Free radicals are "free" because they have an unpaired electron whose purpose is to find a mate. Free radicals can pair up with electrons from other molecules, but they don't do it in a healing or healthful way. The free radicals present in cigarette smoke, pesticides, radiation, toxic chemicals, fried and processed foods, and other unhealthful and unnatural substances simply collide with molecules in the body that have an even number of electrons and steal an electron. The result: More free radicals are born, and the process continues on and on, like a chain reaction.

Free radicals are everywhere, and they constantly attack the body's cells and tissues, unless something is done to stop them. As people get older, these free radicals accumulate, often leading to cancer, arthritis, heart disease, tumors, diabetes, blindness, ulcers—all together more than sixty medical conditions have been associated with free-radical damage. The damage done by free radicals is called "oxidative," the same process that causes metal to rust and our bodies to age. Thus the way to fight the destruction caused by free radicals is with substances that work against ("anti") oxidation—antioxidants.

To visualize how antioxidants work, think about how an apple begins to turn brown after you cut it in half. This is an example of oxidation. To slow the oxidation process, you can coat the cut portion of the fruit with lemon juice, which contains vitamin C. When you eat foods rich in antioxidants, you supply your body with the "lemon juice" it needs to fight free-radical damage.

Which Antioxidants Are the Most Effective?

Scientists have identified dozens of antioxidants, some of which are more·powerful than others, and some which have specific abilities. Below are explanations of the four antioxidants many experts consider to be the most important and the ones often referred to as ACES: vitamins A (as beta-carotene), C, and E, and the mineral selenium. (For information about the many other antioxidants, see Appendix B.)

- *Beta-carotene* is the bright orange pigment that colors a wide variety of fruits and vegetables, from carrots to pumpkins to spinach (although the green chlorophyll dominates the orange in this and many other leafy greens). When you eat foods that contain beta-carotene, your liver converts it into vitamin A. Thus you may hear beta-carotene referred to as provitamin A.

  Beta-carotene neutralizes the harmful effects of tobacco smoke, air pollutants, and other toxins in the environment that can cause cancer. It also appears to hinder the development of skin cancer, early-stage cervical cancer, and cancer of the upper digestive tract. There is significant evidence that beta-carotene helps protect against heart disease and cataracts.

  Common food sources: apricots, broccoli, broccoli sprouts, cantaloupe, carrots, kale, mango, pumpkin, spinach, squash, sweet potatoes

- *Vitamin C* is sometimes called a "super antioxidant" because it is the most powerful antioxidant found in the body. This powerhouse is the only member of this category that is potent enough to stop the oxidants that start free-radical chain reactions. Vitamin C plays a critical role in reducing the risk of cancer, especially the damaging effects of air pollutants, including second-hand smoke.

  Food sources: broccoli, broccoli sprouts, brussels

sprouts, cabbage, cantaloupe, grapefruit juice, honeydew, guava, kale, kiwi, oranges, papaya, red and yellow peppers, potatoes, strawberries, tomatoes

- *Vitamin E* safeguards all the cells in the body from free-radical damage and is particularly protective of vitamins A and C. This antioxidant can protect against cancer as well as cataracts, heart disease, fibrocystic breast disease, leg cramps, stroke, and viral infections.

  Food sources: sunflower seeds, hazelnuts, almonds, sweet potatoes, cottonseed oil, safflower oil, wheat germ, peanut butter, avocados, mangoes, spinach, apricots

- *Selenium* is a potent anticarcinogen and often works closely with vitamin E in the fight against cancer. Yet selenium alone may also be effective as an anticancer agent by blocking tumors and the spread of cancer and by limiting the damage done by toxins that enter the body. Studies suggest that a too low level of selenium in the bloodstream is associated with a greater prevalence of cancer of the breast, colon, rectum, and other body sites.

  Food sources: wheat and rice bran, broccoli, broccoli sprouts, cabbage, celery, cucumbers, garlic, mushrooms, onions, wheat germ, whole-grain flour

PHYTOCHEMICALS

Phytochemicals (*phyto* means "plants") are food components—different from vitamins and minerals—that have the potential to enhance health. While they are in the plant, phytochemicals protect the plant's cells from toxins. When you eat these same plants, the phytochemicals continue to work, but now they are protecting *your* cells. Of the hundreds of phytochemicals researchers have identified (and probably hundreds more yet to be discovered), one many people recognize by name is chlorophyll, the pigment that gives green plants their color.

Researchers still have much to learn about phytochemicals. Because phytochemicals are not necessary for human growth, as vitamins and minerals are, there are no formal standards for how much people need to consume to get the most benefit. Scientists do know, however, that all fruits and vegetables have dozens—even hundreds—of components. Experts believe that it is the combination of elements in a plant—and not a single chemical in any given food—that creates its protective or healing power. As scientists learn more about phytochemicals, it is possible that minimum daily requirements may be set.

The American Dietetic Association tells consumers that phytochemicals are effective in the treatment and/or prevention of cancer, hypertension, diabetes, and cardiovascular disease—all leading causes of death in the United States. Phytochemicals are also important in the prevention and/or treatment of arthritis, osteoporosis, neural tube defects, and bowel dysfunction.

Types of Phytochemicals

There are many classes of phytochemicals, and each one offers some kind of unique protection for the body: protection against cancer-causing substances or invasion by viruses and bacteria, cardiovascular benefits, and so on. To get the most benefit from phytochemicals, it is recommended that you eat a variety of fruits, vegetables, legumes, grains, nuts, and seeds every day.

Here are some of the major phytochemicals that have cancer-fighting capabilities and the foods in which they appear:

- *Bioflavonoids*. More than two hundred plant pigments are in this category. These natural antioxidants are found in tea and wine as well as the peels and skins of fruits and vegetables. Of the more than 1,500 bioflavonoids, some of the more common ones are quercetin (found in grapefruit, red grapes, red and yellow onions, and broccoli, for example), rutin (buckwheat), hesperidin (citrus fruit), and apigenin (chamomile). Overall, bioflavonoids enhance the beneficial effects of vitamin C and help protect against allergies, inflammation, ulcers, viruses, tumors, and other damage from free radicals. They also block the enzymes that produce estrogen, which helps protect against estrogen-induced cancers, and they may also prevent damage to blood vessels.

• *Carotenoids*. Perhaps the best-known nutrient in this class is beta-carotene, a precursor of vitamin A. Carotenoids are the bright orange, red, and yellow pigments that are found in fruits and vegetables such as carrots, grapefruit, tomatoes, cantaloupe, yellow squash, sweet potatoes, pumpkin, and oranges. The carotenoid class contains more than six hundred members. Those like beta-carotene and its relatives—alpha-carotene, epsilon-carotene, gamma-carotene, lycopene, and lutein—protect against cancers of the lung, colon, rectum, breast, uterus, and prostate.

• *Catechins*. These substances are also categorized as bioflavonoids (see above). Catechins are found specifically in black and green teas, and they stop the activity of free radicals involved in the formation of cancer cells.

• *Chlorophyll*. This green pigment is capable of preventing damage to the DNA in cells, which is the first step in the process by which normal cells transform into cancerous ones. Chlorophyll is an antioxidant. It is found in all fruits and vegetables, even those that are not green, as other pigments can mask chlorophyll. Broccoli, brussels sprouts, watercress, spinach, and parsley are excellent sources of chlorophyll.

• *Ellagic Acid*. Ellagic acid works on the front lines by stopping cancer-producing agents from initiating the cancer cell process. It does this in several ways, one of which is to inhibit the activity of carcinogenic compounds that cause DNA damage. Strawberries, cherries, and grapes are the best sources of this substance.

- *Genistein*. Cancer cells need a reliable supply of fresh blood in order to reproduce. The process by which new blood vessels grow around tumors and promote their growth is called angiogenesis. Genistein acts as a road block and stops the flow of blood to tumors. Genistein has even been shown to transform precancerous cells to a healthy state. Soybeans and soy-based foods, such as tofu, soy milk, soy flour, soy-based "meat" products, and miso, are the primary source of this cancer fighter. Among people who traditionally eat soy products, rates of breast, prostate, and uterine cancer are extremely low. Cruciferous vegetables such as brussels sprouts, cabbage, and collards are other good sources of genistein.

- *Glutathione*. This phytochemical is also an antioxidant and is believed to protect the body against various carcinogens, as well as boost overall immune system function. It is found especially in avocados, tomatoes, strawberries, and watermelon.

- *Indoles*. These powerful substances are effective protectants against cancers of the colon, breast, and other sites. They function by allowing detoxification enzymes to form and help the body rid itself of toxins. Many people with fibromyalgia also report symptom relief from eating foods rich in indoles. Indoles are found in cruciferous vegetables such as cabbage, broccoli, broccoli sprouts, brussels sprouts, kale, kohlrabi, mustard greens, rutabaga, turnips, and cauliflower.

- *Lignans*. These agents perform two main functions: They are antioxidants and they disarm estrogen. Both of these actions hinder the growth of certain tumors and protect body cells from carcinogen damage. Lignans are found in seeds and nuts.

- *Limonoids*. Although these specific phytochemicals appear only in the peels and pith of citrus fruit, they have a very important anticancer role: They stimulate the enzymes in the body that detoxify carcinogens. They also protect lung tissue and help clear mucus from the lungs of people with chronic obstructive pulmonary disease. The next time you peel an orange or grapefruit, be sure to leave some of the white pith attached to the sections.

- *Lycopene.* This is the most efficient carotenoid at stopping the free radicals caused by air pollutants and cigarette smoke. It appears to be effective in preventing cancers of the colon and bladder. You'll find lycopene in tomatoes (the best source), guava, watermelon, carrots, and ruby red grapefruit.

- *Monoterpenes.* These phytochemicals have strong antioxidant abilities and also stimulate the enzymes that detoxify cancer-causing substances in the body. Monoterpenes are found in broccoli and its sprouts, cabbage, carrots, eggplant, fruit, parsley, peppers, squash, tomatoes, and yams.

- *Phenols.* Phenols protect against cancer by acting as antioxidants, by neutralizing specific carcinogens, and by promoting the production of natural detoxifying agents in the body. More than two hundred phenols can be found in fruits, potatoes, nuts, garlic, and green tea.

- *Phytoestrogens.* As their name suggests, these substances act like estrogen. They are also known as isoflavones. Phytoestrogens attach themselves to cancer cells and block out the real estrogen the cells need to continue their growth. People who eat foods containing phytoestrogens, such as soy products and beans, are less likely to have breast cancer or to die of pancreatic cancer. See genistein (above) in particular.

- *Phytosterols.* Researchers have studied the seeds of pumpkins, soy beans, rice, and yams and found that phytosterols block the body's ability to absorb cholesterol and aid in excreting it from the body. Phytosterols also appear to block the development of tumors in the colon, prostate, and breast. The highest levels of phytosterols are in the seeds of green and yellow vegetables, although the plants themselves also contain a significant amount.

- *Protease Inhibitors*. These substances perform "strong arm" functions by blocking the spread of cancer cells and limiting the rate at which cancer cells reproduce. Beans, whole grains, soybeans and soy-based foods and beverages are good sources of natural protease inhibitors.

- *Saponins*. These phytochemicals may prevent cancer cells from multiplying. The best sources are soybeans, soybean products, and dried beans. Saponins are also found in spinach, potatoes, tomatoes, and oats.

- *Thiols*. The phytonutrients in this class are found in garlic and the cruciferous vegetables (for example, broccoli, cabbage, and turnips). The cancer fighter sulforaphane is in this category, along with other similar substances that block enzymes that stimulate the growth of tumors in the liver, breast, lung, stomach, esophagus, and colon. To reap this benefit, eat a variety of cruciferous vegetables, as well as onions, leeks, chives, and shallots.

VITAMINS AND MINERALS

In addition to the antioxidant vitamins and nutrients, there are several vitamins and some minerals that can protect against cancer.

B Vitamins

Generally, the vitamins included in this family work closely together and are used by the body for metabolism, the breakdown and use of carbohydrates, fats, and protein for energy. Several of the B vitamins also have a role in strengthening the immune system and thus possess cancer-protection abilities.

Vitamin B_1 (thiamine) works with vitamin B_6 and vitamin E to neutralize free radicals. It can counteract the effects of alcohol and tobacco smoke. Food sources include peanuts, sunflower seeds, bulgur, brewer's yeast, chickpeas, navy beans, brown rice, soybeans, wheat germ, and whole-grain flour.

Vitamin B_2 (riboflavin) teams up with the enzyme glutathione reductase to make another antioxidant, glutathione. Food sources include fortified cereals and breads, broccoli (and its sprouts), spinach, sweet potatoes, and turnip greens.

Vitamin B_3 (niacin/niacinamide) has a key role in metabolism and in maintaining healthy skin, nerves, and mucous membranes. Researchers believe that niacin boosts the cells' ability to resist becoming cancerous. Barley, bulgur, brewer's yeast, beets, peanuts, sunflower seeds, and chicken breast are good sources.

Vitamin B_5 (pantothenic acid) appears to stimulate immune system cells and is important in the manufacture of red blood cells. Whole-grain cereals, nuts, peas, corn, lentils, green leafy vegetables, and mushrooms contain vitamin B_5.

Vitamin B_6 (pyridoxine) is the protein vitamin because it is essential in the manufacture and conversion of protein. Low levels of this vitamin have been associated with a weakened immune system. To prevent this condition, get B_6 from bananas, avocados, carrots, lentils, brown rice, soybeans, sunflower seeds, and whole-grain flour.

Vitamin B_{12} is important in metabolism, in the production of red blood cells, and in maintaining a healthy immune system. This vitamin is found mostly in meat and dairy products, although many cereals and soy products are enriched with vitamin B_{12}. Vitamin B_{12} is also found in sea vegetables and nutritional yeast.

Biotin (or vitamin B_7) is important for a strong immune system. The body manufactures biotin in the intestines and also derives it from foods such as soybeans, oatmeal, bananas, rice bran, barley, and peanut butter.

Folic acid (also known as folacin and folate) is responsible for maintaining cell DNA and a strong immune system.

It also appears to prevent colorectal and cervical cancers by blocking the transformation of normal cells into cancer cells. Excellent sources of folic acid are lentils, black-eyed peas, beans (pinto, adzuki, and black), asparagus, and spinach; chicory, turnip greens, romaine lettuce, avocado, papaya, and parsley are also good sources.

Calcium

Calcium is believed to help reduce the risk of cancer, especially colon cancer. Before you reach for the milk and cheese, consider calcium-rich foods that offer the added bonus of other cancer-fighting phytochemicals. Soy milk and soybean products, legumes, beans, and calcium-rich vegetables (broccoli, broccoli sprouts, collards, spinach, seaweed) can provide all the calcium your body needs while fighting cancer, heart disease, and diabetes. (One cup of cow's milk, fortified soy milk, or fortified rice milk all contain the same amount of calcium, about 280 milligrams.) Whole milk and whole-milk products have been linked to an increased risk of lung cancer and heart disease. Small amounts of low- and nonfat dairy products may be used occasionally but are not considered part of a cancer-prevention diet plan.

Copper

Studies are still ongoing, but scientists have seen evidence that copper slows tumor growth and guards against the harmful effects of radiation, at least in animals. The body uses copper to maintain healthy tissue function and growth, and it works closely with zinc to halt oxidation (see below). Copper is found in navy beans, avocados, nuts and seeds, whole wheat, apricots, and bananas.

Zinc

Zinc is important for maintaining a healthy immune system. It works with copper to neutralize destructive forms of oxygen and also stabilizes cell membranes against damage from carcinogens. Researchers have found a strong correlation between the level of zinc in the prostate and prostate disease. A healthy prostate contains more zinc than any other organ in the human body, and studies of men who have died of this cancer usually show low levels of zinc. Foods with high amounts of zinc include pumpkin seeds, dried beans, lentils, peas, soy products, wheat and rice bran, molasses, sunflower seeds, wheat germ, and whole-grain flour.

FIBER

Your mother or grandmother may have called it "roughage," a term that doesn't make it sound appealing. Fiber is the part of the vegetable, grain, legume, or fruit that, after you eat the food and your body processes it, is not digested. And there are very good reasons, experts believe, why fiber is not destroyed or absorbed during the digestion process. One is that it allows stool to move more quickly through the colon, which reduces the amount of carcinogens and fats in the intestines as well as the amount of time they spend there. This rapid transport process is believed to be a key factor in reducing the risk of colon cancer.

A high-fiber diet is associated with protection against cancers of the esophagus, mouth, pharynx, stomach, and endometrium (lining of the uterus). Fiber also lowers the levels of sex hormones in the body, which prevents or slows the progression of hormone-sensitive cancers such as those of the breast, prostate, and ovaries. There is another anti-cancer property found in vegetable fibers. When vegetable fibers reach the large intestine, fermentation produces a compound called butyrate, which can transform precancerous cells back to normal cells.

Types of Fiber

There are two main types of fiber: water soluble and insoluble. The two kinds of water-soluble fiber are gums and pectins. Gums occur in seeds, oats, and oatmeal and are also added to processed foods. Pectins are found in fruits, vegetables, and seeds, including apples, citrus, dried legumes, lentils, peas, raw cabbage, and strawberries. Water-soluble fiber binds to substances like cholesterol and bile acids, prevents them from being absorbed into the bloodstream, and eliminates some of them in the urine.

Insoluble fiber helps reduce the risk of colon and rectal cancer, and the three types of insoluble fiber include cellulose, lignin, and hemicellulose. Cellulose and lignin are found mostly in whole grains and wheat bran, while hemicellulose occurs in whole grains, nuts, fruits, vegetables, and seeds.

The National Cancer Institute recommends that Americans eat 20 to 30 grams of fiber every day, but most Americans consume about 11 grams or less. If much of your daily fare consists of meat and dairy products, foods made from white flour and/or sugar, and few vegetables, fruits, whole grains, and beans, chances are you are close to the 11-gram mark. Yet according to the National Cancer Institute, if every American ate the recommended amount of fiber, the rate of colon cancer alone could be reduced by 50 percent.

As you increase the amount of fiber in your diet, do it slowly. It may take a week or two for your body to adjust to the increased fiber. During that time you may experience some gas or discomfort in your stomach or intestines. Don't worry; it is only temporary.

Where to Get Fiber

When you add more fruits, vegetables, and whole grains to your diet, you automatically increase the amount of fiber you consume. Center your meals around whole grains and pasta, beans, legumes, rice, vegetables, and fruits rather than meat, poultry, fish, cheese, and milk (all of which contain no fiber). The table below gives the fiber content of some common cancer-fighting foods.

FIBER-RICH FOODS

FOOD	SERVING SIZE	GRAMS FIBER
Fiber One cereal	½ cup	10
Prunes, cooked	½ cup	10
Bran Chex	½ cup	9
Lentils, cooked	½ cup	8
Kidney beans, cooked	½ cup	8
Broccoli, fresh cooked	½ cup	7
Sweet potato, baked	1 small	7
Pita, whole-wheat	1	7
Corn, whole kernel	½ cup	5
Macaroni, whole-wheat	1 cup	5
Pear	1 medium	5
Chickpeas, canned	½ cup	5
Lima beans, cooked	½ cup	5
Beets, pickled	½ cup	4
Apple, w/peel	1 medium	4
Acorn squash, baked	½ cup	4
Peas, green, cooked	½ cup	4
Sauerkraut, canned	½ cup	4
Mango	1 medium	4
Orange	1 medium	4
Tangerine	1 medium	3
Strawberries	1 cup	3
Cantaloupe	1 cup	3
Spinach, cooked	½ cup	3
Cauliflower, cooked	1 cup	3
Rice, brown	½ cup	2
Asparagus, cooked	½ cup	2
Brussels sprouts	½ cup	2
Zucchini, cooked	½ cup	2
Eggplant, cooked	½ cup	2
Carrots, cooked	½ cup	2

ON YOUR PLATE OR IN A PILL?

Popping a pill or two that will provide you with all the phytochemical power you need may sound appealing. However, scientists have found that taking nutrients in supplement form does not provide the disease prevention benefits for which people are looking. The appeal of taking supplements also leaves researchers with unanswered questions, including: What is the optimal amount of each compound? Can phytochemicals be toxic if taken as isolated supplements?

The answer, according to the American Dietetic Association and most nutrition experts, is simple: Increase your consumption of fresh fruits, vegetables, grains, and legumes. Stay away from processed foods. The advantage of getting your nutrients in food rather than in supplements is that the food provides a complete form of nutrition while a supplement offers an isolated component. When you take a vitamin C supplement you get that vitamin only. But when you eat an orange, you absorb vitamin C as well as all the other phytochemicals, nutraceuticals, and fiber it contains—nutrition the way nature intended it to be.

Does this mean nutritional supplements are a waste of time and money? Certainly not. But before you consider taking any supplement, look at your diet. Ideally, food intake should provide complete nutrition. (The menu plans in Chapter 7 are examples of nutritionally well-balanced meals.) However, even people who consume a healthy diet are exposed to factors that affect how well their body assimilates and utilizes the food they eat. Stress (physical, emotional, and environmental), illness, lifestyle choices (smoking, alcohol consumption, use of drugs, amount of sleep), level of exercise, and the quality of food consumed all impact how the body uses the nutrients it takes in. Thus you may need to improve the variety and quality of food you eat, as well as add supplemental vitamins, minerals, and other nutrients and/or herbs to fill in the gaps the diet does not. A nutritionist or other health practitioner can help you plan your supplemental needs.

In this chapter you've learned that there are hundreds, if not thousands, of health-promoting compounds to be found in many foods. In the next chapter you will discover how to build a cancer-prevention eating plan and which foods to include in it.

4. Eat Well and Prosper: Adding Broccoli Sprouts and Other Cancer-Fighting Foods to Your Diet

BY NOW YOU'VE SEEN THAT THERE ARE MANY WAYS TO ENHANCE a cancer-prevention eating plan that includes broccoli sprouts. No one sits down at the dinner table and says, "Now I'm eating phenols, then I'll add some saponin and copper, and for dessert I'll include a dish of pectin." Eating healthy is about eating *food*. That's why in this chapter, the different foods that make up a balanced, low-fat, cancer-fighting eating plan are identified and explained. Some of the questions answered here include: How many broccoli sprouts do you need to eat per day or per week for optimal cancer and disease protection? Which other cancer-preventing foods should you include in your diet? Why are these foods important in the fight against cancer? Which foods and herbal supplements help prevent cancer? Finally, there is a brief review of the latest RDAs (Recommended Daily Allowances) for vitamins and minerals, which are reported by the Food and Drug Administration (FDA) and based on studies conducted by the National Academy of Sciences.

AN OUNCE OF PREVENTION

Research has proved that most of the foods people choose to eat lack essential cancer-preventing nutrients. In fact, many of the foods considered to be standard American fare, such as french fries, hamburgers, hot dogs, pizza, milk shakes, and fried chicken, contain substances that weaken the immune system, making it difficult or impossible for the body to resist cancer and other diseases.

That's where a bit of preventive medicine comes in. In the case of broccoli sprouts, less than one-quarter ounce of prevention a day is all you need. When you include broccoli sprouts as part of a healthful eating plan, you can make a big difference in your health. How much impact can the dietary recommendations mentioned above have on preventing your chances of getting cancer? You be the judge. According to the experts:

- Healthful eating habits could prevent up to 375,000 cases of cancer each year.

- A combination of these dietary choices and not smoking can reduce cancer risk by up to 70 percent.

- A switch to eating five servings of fruits and vegetables a day could lower cancer rates by more than 20 percent.

- Eating a healthful diet, keeping physically active, and maintaining optimal weight can reduce cancer risk by up to 40 percent.

BUILDING A BETTER DIET

To establish a foundation on which you can build a cancer-prevention diet, let's look at a summary of the dietary recommendations offered by the Diet & Cancer Project mentioned in Chapter 1, "Food, Nutrition and the Prevention of Cancer." These recommendations represent the latest research and explain how to construct a balanced diet for cancer and disease prevention and overall good health. None of the guidelines introduces anything new or radical. Yet the fact that they were compiled by a global panel and are the consensus of years of solid research gives you an opportunity to significantly improve your quality of life.

DIETARY RECOMMENDATIONS FROM THE DIET & CANCER PROJECT

Note: All the foods you choose should have undergone little or no processing.

1. Choose a diet that is predominantly plant-based: a variety of fruits, vegetables, legumes, and starches (grains, pasta, breads, and rice).

2. Eat five or more servings of various fruits and vegetables each day (see box below).

3. Eat seven or more servings a day of grains, legumes, roots, tubers, and plantains.

4. Alcohol is not recommended. Limit the amount per day to one drink if you are a woman, and two if you are a man.

5. Red meat is not recommended. Limit to less than 3 ounces per day. If you do eat animal protein, choose fish or chicken without the skin and prepare it without added fat (broil, poach, steam, or bake).

6. Limit consumption of fatty foods, especially those made from animals, such as dairy items. Use vegetable oils in moderation, and consider healthier oils such as olive oil.

7. Avoid eating any food that has been charred or burned. A one-pound steak cooked over charcoal has as much benzopyrene (a carcinogen) as six hundred cigarettes.

8. Limit consumption of table salt and salty foods. Instead, use spices and herbs to season food.

9. Properly store perishable foods.

Although not related directly to diet, two other recommendations that made the list are worth mentioning: exercise every day, especially if your daily activity level is low or moderate; and avoid all tobacco products, both smoking and chewing. (For a free brochure about the report, see Appendix B.)

HOW MUCH IS ONE SERVING?

FRUITS AND VEGETABLES

- 1/2 cup cooked or chopped raw fruit or vegetable
- 1 cup raw leafy vegetable
- 1 medium piece of fruit
- 1/4 cup dried fruit
- 6 ounces vegetable or fruit juice

PROTEIN (SOY, LEGUMES, DAIRY, MEAT)

- 1/2 cup cooked dried beans or legumes
- 2 tablespoons nut butter (peanut, almond, sesame)
- 2 to 3 ounces lean meat, fish, or poultry
- 2 ounces soy-based meat substitute products
- 1/2 cup soy milk
- 1 1/2 ounces tofu
- 1 egg
- handful of seeds or nuts (unsalted)
- 1 cup cow's milk (low or nonfat)
- 1 1/2 ounces natural cheese (low or nonfat)

BREAD, CEREALS, PASTA, RICE

- 1 slice bread
- 1 ounce dry cereal
- 1/2 cup cooked pasta, rice, grain
- 1/2 bagel or English muffin
- 3 to 4 plain crackers

A BALANCED, HEALTHFUL FOOD PLAN

In the early 1990s, the U.S. Department of Agriculture (USDA) had plans to revise the old food pyramid and incorporate more healthful, disease-preventing guidelines. Under pressure from the meat and dairy industries, however, they changed their plans to reduce recommended meat and dairy food. Thus the resulting new food pyramid does not meet cancer-prevention, disease-fighting guidelines and needs some modifications.

The modified food pyramid, reflects the latest recommendations from the Cancer Institute, which places more emphasis on low-fat, cancer-fighting, high-protein vegetable foods than does the USDA version. This modified version allows for small amounts of animal protein for those who have not eliminated meat (as recommended by the Cancer Institute and many other health experts) and dairy products from their diet, as well as portions of fish. (For a food pyramid that was created specifically to prevent and fight cancer, as well as diabetes and heart disease, see *Permanent Remissions*, by Robert Haas; also see *Save Yourself From Breast Cancer*, by Robert M. Kradjian, M.D., and other books in Appendix B.)

Let's look at the elements of the modified pyramid, from the bottom up.

Grains, Cereals, Roots, Tubers, Plantains

The minimum recommended servings in this category are seven. It is easy to mix and match menu items from the many entries in this group. The menu plans and recipes in Chapter 7 show you how.

Grains and Cereals. Whole grains and cereals are excellent sources of phytochemicals, vitamins (especially B and E), minerals (iron, magnesium, and zinc), fiber, and protein. They contain very little fat and no cholesterol. To maximize mineral absorption, eat a vitamin C source with your whole grains. This is easy to do: Whole-grain pasta and marinara sauce, Fruity French Toast (recipe in Chapter 7), or drinking vegetable or fruit juice with a meal that includes grains are just a few ways to accomplish this.

Look for whole-grain products, such as breads, bagels, crackers, flours, muffins, pasta, and air-popped popcorn; brans (rice, oat, and wheat); and germs (wheat and rice). Both the brans and germs of grains can be added to recipes for muffins and breads, or sprinkled on your cereal or casseroles to add both nutrients and fiber to your diet. Avoid white bread and other overprocessed baked goods. Whole-grain products can be made from any one or more of the following varieties of grains:

- **Amaranth:** A very high-protein grain that is used as a side dish and in salads, or popped like popcorn.

- **Barley:** Use as a hot cereal and in soups, cold salads, and pilafs.

- **Buckwheat:** Not really wheat at all, so it can be eaten by people who are allergic to wheat. Buckwheat is very high in protein and is often used in breads and pancakes.

- **Corn:** A versatile grain that comes in many forms: sweet corn, popcorn, polenta, grits, corn pastas, hominy, and masa harina (ground hominy used to make tortillas and corn chips).

- **Kamut:** Use in hot and cold grain salads and as a cereal.

- **Millet:** Use in casseroles, stews, soups, and muffins, and as a cereal.

- **Oats:** Usually used as a cereal; forms include rolled oats, quick oats, oat bran, and oat groats.

- **Quinoa:** This grain has the highest protein level of all the grains. Use it in stews, stuffing, breads, and soups.

- **Rice:** Varieties include arborio, basmati, brown, jasmine, Texamati, and wehani.

- **Triticale:** A hybrid cross between wheat and rye, which makes it more nutritious than either grain alone. It can be bought as whole berries, flakes, or flour. Use it in casseroles and salads and as a cereal.

• Wheat: Comes in several forms: wheat berries (use as a cereal or as a side dish); bulgur (make taboule); couscous (as a side dish); and semolina (wheat pasta). The gluten can be stripped from the wheat and made into a high-protein meat substitute called seitan.

• Roots, Tubers, and Plantains: Foods in this category include potatoes, yams, sweet potatoes, carrots, turnips, beets, rutabaga, parsnips, and kohlrabi. Use cooked or raw in salads.

Vegetables

In this category are vegetables generally not included in the "Roots, Tubers, Plantains" group above, although a few do cross over. For optimal cancer protection, include the following vegetables in your daily menu plans and make sure you eat at least three different "colors" per day:

• *Cruciferous*, at least two servings daily: beet greens, bok choy, broccoli, broccoli sprouts, brussels sprouts, cabbage, cauliflower, collard greens, kale, kohlrabi, mustard greens, radish, rutabaga, turnip greens, and turnips

• *Antioxidant*-rich veggies, one to two servings daily: tomatoes, bell peppers (red, green, and yellow), asparagus, spinach, squash (winter and summer)

• *Leafy Greens*, one to two servings daily: sprouts (broccoli, alfalfa, mung bean, and others), escarole, chicory, dandelion greens, sorrel, Swiss chard, dark green lettuce (loose leaf, romaine, butter)

• *Other Vegetables*, one serving daily: mushrooms, sea vegetables (kelp, agar-agar, dulse, carrageenan, nori, wakame, kombu), green beans, cucumbers, pumpkin, okra, water chestnuts

Fruits

Incorporate two to four servings daily of fruit, including at least one citrus (orange, grapefruit, tangerine, lemon). One serving can be a fruit juice; the remaining should be whole fruits because they include fiber, which is generally lost in juicing. Fresh, dried, and stewed fruits are included in this group.

Dairy, Soy Items, Beans/Legumes, Nuts, Meat, Fish

This is a broad category that contains much of the protein foods. The Cancer Institute recommends that you get most, if not all, of your protein from nonanimal sources. Choose from the following options:

• *Dairy.* If choosing dairy products, select up to one serving per day of a low-fat or nonfat milk, yogurt, or cheese.

• *Beans/Legumes.* Two servings per day, one of which can be soy foods. Choose from beans (adzuki, black, black-eyed peas, brown, pinto, red, fava, lima, kidney, navy, white, chickpeas), lentils, split peas, and green peas.

• *Soy Foods.* If you haven't tried a soy burger or soy "hot dog" recently, you may be in for a pleasant surprise. As competition among a growing number of soy food and beverage manufacturers has grown, the taste, texture, and variety of these products have improved dramatically. Soy-based meat and dairy substitutes are available in the form of hamburger, sausage, bacon, turkey and pastrami slices, chicken, ground beef, soy milk and soy cheese, yogurt, and frozen desserts. (See Appendix A for manufacturers.) Also in this category are textured vegetable protein (TVP), tofu, tempeh, miso, soy nuts, soy flour, and soy grits.

• *Meat and Fish.* Avoid all beef, pork, organ meats,

and any other smoked, cured, or processed meat products. If you do include meat or fish in your diet, limit your servings to 3 ounces or less, three to five times a week, of skinless poultry or fish.

You've probably heard a lot about how good fish is for you, but there is a caveat. According to Andrew Weil, M.D., author of *Natural Health, Natural Medicine, 8 Weeks to Optimum Health*, and several other best-selling health books, only specific fish are recommended. Oily, cold-water fish—salmon, kippers, mackerel, and sardines—are rich in omega-3 oils, help reduce the risk of heart attack, and improve blood fat levels. Freshwater fish, shellfish, and most large ocean fish (including tuna) are contaminated with various known carcinogens and other toxic substances and may not be safe for human consumption.

• *Nuts and Seeds.* One handful of nuts and/or seeds several times a week provides an excellent source of protein and fiber without cholesterol. Enjoy them unsalted, roasted, or raw, or as a spread. Most nut and seed butters are recommended (tahini, sesame, hazelnut, walnut, almond, cashew, and sunflower butters). A notable exception is peanut butter, which contains high levels of aflatoxins, which can be carcinogenic when consumed in large quantities. Limit to about 4 tablespoons per week. Eat nuts as a snack or add them to casseroles, salads, or vegetables. Nut butters can be used to make a quick, nutritious sandwich.

Fats, Oils, and Sweets

Up to one serving per day of fats and oils is recommended. The best oils to use for cooking or salad dressing are canola, olive, and nut oils (walnut, almond, and macadamia). Soy-based mayonnaise also is an option for salad dressing.

The average American consumes more than two pounds of sugar every week, and a link between sugar consumption and cancer has been found. Researchers in Italy have linked sugar use with an increased risk of rectal and colon cancers, while experts in the Netherlands found a similar association between sugar and gallbladder and biliary tract cancers.

Limit sweets to 1 tablespoon of added sweetener per day, such as syrup, molasses, honey, sugar, jelly, and jams. Try to get your "sweet fix" from the natural sugars found in fruit. Beware of "hidden" sugar in products such as ready-to-eat cereals (both sweetened and unsweetened), baked goods, soda, fruit beverages (not juices), sauces, and gravies. A more recent area of concern regarding added sugar is in low-fat and no-fat baked goods and snacks. Read the labels on these products. Although they may contain little or no significant fat, the general practice is to add more sugar to the product to make up for the taste that is lost by removing the fat.

A Few Words About Fat

In *Save Yourself From Breast Cancer*, by Robert M. Kradjian, M.D., his breast cancer prevention plan calls for reducing total dietary fat intake to no more than 20 percent of total calories, while 10 percent is optimal. Dr. Kradjian specifically recommends that people avoid all dairy products, eliminate or dramatically reduce intake of animal proteins, and avoid all hydrogenated oils and instead use seed oils. In Dr. Kradjian's opinion, "The data support a link between increased use of vegetable oils and hydrogenated fats with the increase in breast cancer rates. In the 1960's, when the association between saturated fat, cholesterol, and heart disease was established, we radically increased our intake of vegetable oils and hydrogenated fats in an attempt to escape coronary artery disease." The result is that Americans now consume more than 21 pounds of these oils every year, a change that Dr. Kradjian believes has had a "massive negative impact on our health." It appears that in an attempt to protect the heart by reducing intake of saturated fats, we have "caused increases in breast, prostate, and colon cancers."

The high incidence of prostate cancer among American

men also has been linked to fat consumption, specifically the saturated fat found in red meat. Comparison studies have been conducted of breast and prostate cancer rates among people in Japan and other countries where deaths from these cancers are rare and among immigrants from these countries who have adopted the American diet. The immigrants' chances of developing these cancers eventually equal those of native-born Americans. Some researchers believe that the increase in fat consumption is the reason for the rise in cancer incidence; others say it's the decline in consumption of cancer-protective foods, such as soybeans, soybean-based products, and green tea. These foods have phytoestrogens that block the tumor-making abilities of the hormones estrogen and testosterone.

While the fat and cancer debate continues, scientists do know that when it comes to the number-one killer in America—heart disease—fat consumption plays a major role. Controlling dietary fat is also important in diabetes, hypertension, arthritis, and various gastrointestinal disorders.

CULINARY CANCER FIGHTERS

The modified food pyramid is a general dietary plan that encourages you to eat a wide variety of foods. Now let's look at specific foods in that plan that help safeguard against cancer. Fortunately, there are many anticancer foods—yet not all of them are effective in the same way. Some, like broccoli sprouts and other cruciferous vegetables, contain anticancer compounds such as chlorophyll and carotenoids. Foods high in fiber, such as whole grains, protect the body from contact with cancer-causing agents, especially in the intestines. Others are high in antioxidants, which guard the cells against damage from free radicals.

Top-ten lists are popular, but presenting you with the top ten cancer-fighting foods would be a great disservice because there are so many more that can help you fight this disease. That's why the following list has more than fifty of the best cancer-protective foods. Included are recommendations from the National Cancer Institute, the Cancer Treatment Institutes of America, and the American Cancer Institute, and from experts such as Barry Fox, Ph.D., Andrew Weil, M.D., Robert Haas, M.S., and others. These foods form the basis of the recipes in Chapter 7. With a list this long and varied, you can't get bored and you'll never go hungry. And you'll be

TOP CANCER-PROTECTIVE FOODS

Apples	Mangoes
Apricots	Mushrooms
Asparagus	Nuts (most varieties)
Avocados	Oats
Barley	Onions
Beans (all varieties)	Oranges
Broccoli and its sprouts	Papaya
Brussels sprouts	Parsley
Cabbage	Pasta
Cantaloupe	Peppers
Carrots	Potatoes
Cauliflower	Pumpkin
Celery	Radishes
Collard greens	Rice (especially brown)
Currants	Sea vegetables
Dandelion greens	Seeds
Eggplant	Spinach
Figs	Strawberries
Flaxseed	Tangerines
Garlic	Tea
Grapes	Tofu (and other soy foods)
Grapefruit	Tomatoes
Guava	Turnips
Kale	Watercress
Kiwi	Watermelon
Lemons	Wheat
Lentils	

providing your body with the gift of health, because most of these foods protect not only against cancer but also other serious diseases, such as heart disease, hypertension, diabetes, cataracts, osteoporosis, and arthritis, among others.

Let's take a closer look at some of these items and see what special qualities make them potent cancer-fighting foods.

• *Apples.* Fruit contains anticancer substances known as phenols, which neutralize certain carcinogens, disrupt the transformation of precancerous cells into cancerous ones, and stimulate the body's production of natural cancer fighters. Apples also contain a soluble fiber called pectin, which is known to reduce the risk of colon cancer. Most of the pectin is in the peel, so it is best to buy organically grown apples, or thoroughly wash conventionally grown apples before eating.

• *Apricots.* These small fruits are good sources of betacarotene, vitamin C, and fiber. The antioxidants betacarotene and vitamin C help strengthen the body's immune system against cancerous agents and their damage to the cells, while the fiber helps dilute carcinogens in the intestines and move them more quickly out of the body. Include fresh or dried apricots in your diet as a dessert or snack.

• *Asparagus.* This plant was called the "king of vegetables" by the ancient Romans and Greeks, who used it to treat arthritis, toothache, and infertility. Today researchers know it contains the potent antioxidant glutathione, which is helpful in the fight against cancer, cataracts, and heart disease.

• *Avocados.* The avocado is an excellent source of the antioxidant glutathione and a good source of vitamins C and B_6. Although high in calories and fat, the fat is the "good" kind—the monounsaturated fat found in olive oil. Because of its high fat content, include avocados less often in your diet than other fruits, perhaps once or twice a week.

• *Barley.* This grain's high fiber content makes it effective in reducing the risk of cancer of the colon, rectum, pancreas, prostate, and breast. The protease inhibitors in barley prevent the development of cancer by stopping carcinogenic agents from attaching themselves to the intestinal walls.

• *Beans.* These powerhouses of nutrition are also versatile in the kitchen. They contain good amounts of protease inhibitors, lignans, phytoestrogens, and fiber—all potent cancer fighters. Studies show that people who make beans a significant part of their diet are less likely to have breast cancer or to die of pancreatic cancer.

The many varieties of beans (see "Beans/Legumes," page 46) can be prepared in many ways, including hot in soups, chili, casseroles, and salads; cold in dips, salads, and sandwich spreads; and sprouted. To eliminate the intestinal gas beans are known to cause, rinse the raw beans, soak them in water for at least one hour, discard the water, and cook the beans in fresh water. Adding a few cloves of garlic or pieces of ginger to the cooking water also decreases the tendency for gas formation.

• *Broccoli Sprouts, Broccoli, and Other Cruciferous Vegetables.* Although some of the vegetables in this group may appear to have nothing in common (for example, radishes and bok choy), their association lies in the fact that all of these plants have pointed pods and cross-shaped ("crucifer") flowers. In addition, all of the cruciferous vegetables contain the powerful anticancer agents sulforaphane (see Chapters 1 and 2) and indole-3-carbinol (see Chapter 3), with broccoli sprouts leading the way in cancer-prevention power. Include at least one vegetable, preferably two, from this group every day, and make one of them broccoli sprouts.

• *Cantaloupe.* Just one-half cantaloupe contains 186 percent of the RDA for vitamin C and nearly 90 percent for vitamin A—two powerful antioxidants that help fight cancer. Eat it often when it's in season.

• *Carrots.* One medium carrot has more than 200 percent of the RDA of vitamin A, an antioxidant that is known to fight cancers of the esophagus, bladder, larynx, lung, prostate, cervix, neck, head, and stomach. Carrots also contain the cancer fighters p-coumaric acid and chloregenic acid (also in strawberries) and the powerful antioxidant lycopene, found in abundance in tomatoes.

• *Celery.* Many people think of celery as a boring diet food, yet it contains several powerful anticancer agents, such as phthalides and polyacetylenes. These substances render carcinogens harmless, before they have the opportunity to cause damage. Studies suggest celery is particularly effective against stomach cancer.

• *Currants.* Black currants contain more than 300 percent of the RDA for vitamin C, while the red and white varieties contain nearly 80 percent. This makes black currants especially effective in protecting against cancers of the stomach, pancreas, cervix, rectum, breast, lungs, and esophagus. All varieties of currants contain flavonoids, which help the body resist carcinogens. Currants are not always readily available in the produce aisle, so you may have to ask the produce or store manager for them. Note: If you have kidney stones or a tendency to develop them, avoid currants, as they contain oxalic acid.

• *Eggplant.* This vegetable comes in several varieties, most commonly purple and white. Eggplant contains significant amounts of terpenes and other cancer-fighting phytochemicals and is a good low-fat, low-calorie addition to any diet. Because it can absorb a lot of oil, it is best to bake, steam, broil, or boil this vegetable.

• *Figs.* Japanese researchers have used injections and oral formulas of fig extracts to shrink tumors in cancer patients. You don't need to go to that length to enjoy the cancer-fighting properties of figs. You can include a few fresh or dried figs in your diet each week, as they are a good source of natural sweetness. Dried figs, however, are high in sugar and calories, so you may want to limit the amount you eat.

• *Flaxseed.* A type of fiber called lignan in flaxseed appears to disrupt the development of tumors of the breast, colon, rectum, prostate, and other sites. Flaxseeds can be used as an egg substitute in baking, or tossed into a stir-fry to add a nutty taste. Flaxseed flour or meal can be added to recipes for breads, muffins, cookies, and other baked goods.

• *Garlic and Onions.* Chemicals called allylic sulfides, present in significant amounts in garlic and onions and somewhat less in leeks, chives, and shallots, are believed to stimulate enzymes in the body that neutralize cancer-causing substances.

Garlic contains more than thirty substances known to help fight cancer, including ajoene, quercetin, and diallyl sulfide. Studies of both people and animals show that eating garlic—and onions—lowers the rates of breast, colon, and esophageal cancers.

Onions contain about 150 phytochemicals, and researchers have discovered that the phytochemicals consisting of sulfur compounds have antioxidant powers and appear to reverse some of the cancer-causing cell damage performed by free radicals. Yellow and red onions (but not white) contain high amounts of quercetin, which defuses cancer-causing agents and enzymes that stimulate cancer growth, especially stomach cancer. For optimal cancer protection, include one-half onion and three cloves of garlic to your diet per day.

• *Grapes.* Like strawberries, grapes contain ellagic acid, a powerful inhibitor of cancer cell growth. The antioxidant quercetin is found in red grapes, and extracts of Concord grapes retard tumor growth in animals. European grapes (Thompson) have higher levels of vitamin C and fiber than their American cousins.

• *Guava, Mango, and Papaya.* All three of these tropical fruits are excellent sources of the cancer-fighting antioxidant vitamin C: guava, 275 percent of RDA; mango, 90 percent; and papaya, 317 percent. For cancer-fighting fiber in the form of pectin, guava has the greatest amount (4.5 grams), with mangoes and papayas not far behind. Studies show a 50 percent reduction in the rate of colon cancer among animals fed pectin. Include one or all of these tropical fruits in your menu plan when they are in season.

• *Kiwi.* The kiwi hails from China, where it was traditionally used to treat cancer. Its high vitamin C content (124 percent of RDA per serving) and significant amount of fiber make it a good menu choice in the fight against cancer. Include several per week when they are in season.

• *Lentils.* A single serving of this legume contains 86 percent of the RDA for folic acid, an important anticancer vitamin. Other cancer-fighting substances in lentils are phytates, which help hinder the development of cancer; and fiber, which protects against colon, rectal, pancreatic, prostate, and breast cancers.

• *Mushrooms.* The medicinal value of mushrooms is found not in the button variety, but in the more exotic reishi, shiitake, and maitake. These mushrooms stimulate the T cells in the immune system, which appear to have effective cancer-fighting abilities. Shiitake contain a powerful antitumor agent called lentinan, while an anticancer agent called beta-glucan has been found in maitake.

Anticancer drugs extracted from these and other exotic mushrooms have been approved by the Japanese equivalent of the FDA and are used throughout Europe and Japan. Reishi, shiitake, and maitake mushrooms have become more available in the U.S. in mainstream supermarkets. They can be purchased either fresh or dried for addition to casseroles, soups, stews, stir-fries, and salads.

• *Nuts.* Nuts are a good source of fiber, magnesium, and protease inhibitors, the latter of which disrupt the activity of enzymes that stimulate cancer growth. Different nuts possess different anticancer abilities. For example,

Brazil nuts are rich in selenium, which is associated with lower cancer risk. Oleic acid and ellagic acid, which may protect against cancer, are in walnuts. The cancer-preventive mineral magnesium is found in almonds, filberts, hickory nuts, and cashews. All nuts except chestnuts are high in fat, so use them sparingly as a substitute for meat, poultry, dairy, and other fatty foods. Note: Because nuts contain high levels of the amino acid arginine, people with herpes should avoid nuts.

• *Oats.* Known for their ability to lower cholesterol, whole oats and oat bran are important in preventing cancer. Both contain phytates, substances that may disrupt cancer development by disengaging the hormones that encourage tumor growth. Include oatmeal and/or oat bran in your menu several times a week.

• *Oranges and Other Citrus Fruits.* When it comes to cancer-fighting power, oranges are near the top of the list. They contain every type of natural anticancer substance scientists have discovered to date. Oranges, grapefruit, tangerines, lemons, and limes contain more than fifty substances that fight cancer, including antioxidants, flavonoids, terpenes, limonoids, and carotenoids. Monoterpenes, for example, remove carcinogens (such as those from air pollution, food, or smoke) from cells to prevent them from becoming cancerous.

Citrus fruits are also excellent sources of vitamin C: just one orange or grapefruit supplies more than 100 percent of the Recommended Daily Allowance of this cancer-fighting vitamin. While studying the protective effects of vitamin C against cancer, researchers made an interesting discovery: 3 ounces of freshly squeezed orange juice per day are more effective than a supplement containing 1,000 milligrams of vitamin C, even though the juice contains only 40 milligrams of the vitamin. Additional studies were done with the same result. Clearly, oranges contain other cancer-fighting phytochemicals, and they all work together to produce the beneficial effect.

If you want to significantly reduce your risk of developing pancreatic cancer, eat a grapefruit every day.

• *Parsley.* Ounce for ounce, parsley has more vitamin C than carrots and sweet potatoes and more beta-carotene than broccoli or spinach. Parsley also contains other anticancer substances, including flavonoids, polyacetylenes, coumarins, chlorophyll, and monoterpenes. Add several sprigs to your menu daily. It freshens your breath, too!

• *Pasta.* Pasta's anticancer power lies in its fiber content. If you eat the whole-wheat varieties, you'll get the maximum effect: Whole-grain versions have more than double the fiber of other pastas. When served with tomato sauce and/or vegetables, beans, or legumes, you have a delicious, cancer-fighting meal. Enjoy it several times a week.

• *Peppers.* Both hot chili peppers and sweet peppers are high in antioxidants; in fact, one chili pepper has 200 percent of the RDA for vitamin C and 100 percent of RDA for beta-carotene. Sweet green peppers also contain the anticancer agents p-coumaric acid and chloregenic acid (as do strawberries), and sweet red peppers contain lycopene, the potent cancer fighter found in tomatoes.

• *Potatoes.* White potatoes and sweet potatoes are both good sources of the antioxidant vitamin C, while sweet potatoes have an exceptional amount of vitamin A. Potatoes also contain the anticancer agents polyphenols and protease inhibitors, which help prevent the development of cancerous cells. Include these tubers daily, if possible.

• *Pumpkin.* The two anticancer ingredients most prominent in pumpkin are beta-carotene and fiber. A one-half cup serving of pumpkin contains 250 percent of the RDA for beta-carotene and 3.4 grams of fiber. Pumpkin has the distinction of being served in just about any course of a meal: pumpkin soup, pumpkin bread, as a vegetable side dish, or as a dessert in pie or custard.

• *Rice.* Brown rice is the anticancer favorite when compared to white rice. One-half cup of brown rice contains 67 percent of the RDA for thiamine. Low levels of thiamine have been linked with an increased risk of prostate cancer. Rice also is a source of protease inhibitors and fiber.

• *Sea Vegetables.* Fuciodan is the name of the anti-cancer ingredient in sea vegetables (or seaweeds) that helps prevent the development of cancer and slows the rate of the disease if it is already present. Sea vegetables such as kelp, nori, sea lettuce, dulse, and Irish moss can be added to stews, soups, and casseroles, or rolled around rice to create nori rolls.

• *Seeds.* Seeds are the single most important food source for humans: More than 60 percent of the protein consumed in the world comes from seeds. Although beans, grains, lentils, and peas are seeds, they have been covered elsewhere. The seeds discussed here are specific types, such as sunflower, pumpkin, and sesame. These foods contain protease inhibitors, which help to hinder cancer growth and also act as antioxidants. Sesame seed, for example, contains sesamin, an antioxidant that helps counteract cancer processes in the body. Pumpkin seeds contain high amounts of zinc and are used to guard against and treat prostate cancer. Because of their high caloric and fat content, use seeds as a condiment, sprinkled on cereal, casseroles, or salads, or as an occasional light snack.

• *Soybean-Based Foods.* A diet rich in soybeans and soy-based foods (tempeh, tofu, textured vegetable protein [TVP], miso, soy milk, and meat and dairy analogues) appears to offer protection against cancer and cardiovascular disease. One reason for this benefit is the presence of substances called isoflavones, which are chemically similar to estrogen and testosterone. The isoflavones block the action of these two hormones and thus the development of breast and prostate cancers, which are hormone-sensitive. Large studies conducted in Asia, where people eat a diet high in soybeans, show that soybeans can nearly eliminate the threat of some cancers, such as breast, cervical, and prostate cancers.

Soybeans also contain other cancer-fighting phyto-chemicals. Genistein, for example, inhibits the enzymes used by cancer cells for growth. Other phytochemicals include phytic acid, protease inhibitors, saponins, and sugars known as fruto-oligosaccharides.

Researchers note that although soybeans are beneficial for people who eat a low-fat diet, the advantages may not be maintained for people who consume high-fat foods.

• *Spinach.* This leafy green vegetable is rich in folic acid, a potent anticancer vitamin (see page 33).

• *Strawberries.* This berry contains several cancer-fighting substances. High on the list is vitamin C: One cup of strawberries has 141 percent of the RDA for this vitamin, which helps the components of the immune system destroy cancerous growths. A high level of ellagic acid, a proven cancer-fighter, is also found in this fruit. Two other substances in strawberries, p-coumaric acid and chloregenic acid, help reduce the risk of cancer by attaching themselves to cancer-causing nitric oxides from certain foods and flushing them out of the body. Finally, the fiber in strawberries helps protect against cancers of the colon, pancreas, breast, prostate, and rectum.

Because strawberries are typically heavily treated with pesticides, buy only organically grown strawberries. Enjoy them fresh, frozen, or cooked: Ellagic acid contin-ues to offer its cancer protection despite extreme changes in temperature.

• *Tea.* Green tea may help reduce the incidence of can-cers of the esophagus, lung, stomach, and skin. The ingre-dients that may be responsible for this cancer-fighting ability are powerful antioxidants and bioflavonoids called catechins (see Chapter 3), and one catechin in particular: epigallocatechin gallate. Green tea also contains vitamins A, C, and E. Although most of the research on the bene-fits of green tea has been done in animals, results of sev-eral studies in humans suggest that drinking green tea significantly lowers the risk of developing cancers of the pancreas, stomach, colon, and esophagus. In 1994, the National Cancer Institute reported that green tea could reduce the incidence of esophageal cancer. Hot or cold (and preferably naturally decaffeinated), tea is a good beverage choice.

• *Tomatoes.* Who can resist a juicy, plump tomato plucked from the vine? Pick with abandon, because tomatoes have a special antioxidant called lycopene, which is believed to be more powerful than beta-carotene when it comes to fighting certain free radicals. Lycopene's specific ability is helping reduce the risk of cervical, colon, pancreatic, stomach, rectal, oral, pharynx, and esophageal cancers. Include tomatoes and tomato products in your diet daily if possible.

• *Watermelon.* Like tomatoes, watermelon contains the powerful anticancer antioxidant called lycopene. Watermelon also is a good source of vitamin C. Enjoy it several times a week when it is in season.

• *Wheat.* The many faces of wheat—wheat berries, wheat bran, groats, cracked wheat, couscous—offer a good source of fiber and a reduced risk of colon cancer. Wheat also lowers the level of estrogen in the blood, which reduces the risk of breast and prostate cancers. One more feature of wheat is the presence of ferulic acid, which has demonstrated anticancer abilities in lab animals.

This list of culinary cancer fighters is proof of the many options available to you and others to ward off cancer and other serious diseases. As promised, the choices are varied, and you're sure to find many foods you can include as a regular part of your diet.

SUPPLEMENTS FOR CANCER PROTECTION

If you have a car or house or something else of great value, you probably take good care of it. After all, it's an investment.

So it's likely that you also carry an insurance policy on those possessions, just in case something unforeseen happens.

Food and herbal supplements are something like that: a little additional peace of mind for your most valued possession, your health. They should be viewed as added protection, not as a "cure all." Preventing disease is far less expensive than treatment. So even if you follow a healthy lifestyle most of the time, but especially if you don't, you may want to take supplements as an additional hedge against cancer. (Note: Please consult with your physician before starting *any* supplement program.)

Astragalus

Also known as milk vetch root, astragalus is used in both Western and Chinese medicines to stimulate the immune system. It is believed to help increase the number of antibodies in the body, which in turn boosts the body's ability to destroy toxins and other foreign invaders. In people with cancer, astragalus may increase immune system response two- to threefold. Astragalus is available as a prepared tea or fluid extract, or in capsules. It is not known to cause side effects and can be taken daily as an immune system booster.

Asian Ginseng

Regular consumption of Asian ginseng (*Panax ginseng*) may protect against cancer. The most effective forms of ginseng are the extract and the powder. If you take a supplement, buy ginseng that has been standardized by its ginsenoside content, and take it according to package directions.

Berberine

Berberine is a type of alkaloid that is found in several herbs, notably goldenseal, barberry, Oregon grape, and goldthread. Studies conducted in laboratories using animal and human cancer cells indicate that berberine kills existing tumor cells, but whether berberine is effective in protecting the body against the development of cancer has not been determined. It is effective, however, in raising the white blood cell levels of people with cancer who are undergoing chemotherapy or radiation. A standard dosage of goldenseal is ½ to 1 teaspoon of fluid extract, three times a day. Higher dosages may disrupt vitamin B metabolism.

Dong Quai

Dong quai belongs to the *Angelica* species of herbs that are grown throughout the United States, Europe, and Asia. Dong quai is most often used to treat "female disorders" because it has highly active phytoestrogens. Dong quai helps balance estrogen levels in the body. This characteristic also makes it useful as an indirect preventive measure for cancers of the uterus and breast, which are hormone-driven cancers. Dong quai also contains various coumarins, which have the ability to destroy cancer cells. A typical dosage of dong quai is 1 to 2 grams of powdered root—either in a capsule or as a tea— three times a day, or 1 teaspoon of tincture three times a day.

Omega-3 Fatty Acids

This natural substance, found in flaxseed, canola oil, hempseed oil, salmon, and mackerel, inhibits the development of tumors in animals and helps halt the progress of cell growth in human and animal cells in the laboratory. It also helps precancerous cells transform back to normal cells and hinders the growth of blood vessels in cancer cells. A protective amount of omega-3 can be gotten from 1 to 2 tablespoons of ground flaxseed per week, added to salads, soups, or other foods, or from one serving of salmon per week.

Saw Palmetto

The berries of this herb are used throughout Europe to treat benign prostatic hyperplasia—enlargement of the prostate gland. The berries contain a fatty acid that prevents the creation of DHT, the compound that is believed to be involved in the development of prostate cancer. The usual dose is 160 milligrams, twice a day, of the standardized extract.

Turmeric

Turmeric (*Curcuma longa*) is a member of the ginger family of herbs. This perennial contains a substance called curcumin, which has anticancer properties. You may recognize turmeric as being the primary ingredient in curry powder. Besides its culinary appeal, turmeric and the extract curcumin have demonstrated power against the formation and progression of cancer. They also appear to suppress the damaging actions of carcinogens such as cigarette smoke, while turmeric boosts the body's antioxidant abilities.

Turmeric is not a commonly used herb, so in addition to adding it to your diet you may want to take a supplement. As a supplement, turmeric is usually taken in the form of a curcumin-bromelain combination to allow maximum absorption. Look for combinations that include 400 to 600 milligrams of curcumin and take the supplement up to three times a day on an empty stomach.

VITAMIN/MINERAL SUPPLEMENTS: DO YOU NEED THEM?

If you eat a healthful, balanced diet, a daily multivitamin and mineral pill may not be necessary. However, many physicians believe it is a good insurance policy because there are many factors that can negatively affect the nutritional value of the food you eat or, once eaten, prevent optimal use by your body. Some of these factors include the following:

• *Food preparation.* Peeling fruits and vegetables removes much of their vitamin, mineral, and fiber content. Eating organic produce is one way to eliminate the need to peel your food (see Chapter 5). Also, steaming and stir-frying vegetables helps preserve their nutritional value, while boiling, frying, and overcooking depletes nutrients.

• *Soil.* Again, organic produce is the better choice, because not only has it not been treated with toxic chemicals, but the soil in which it is grown is richer in the nutrients the plant needs to grow and thus to pass along to those who eat it.

• *Freshness.* How fresh is the produce you buy? Storage time has a significant impact on the nutritional value of fruits and vegetables (see Chapter 5).

The following list of nutrients and their recommended doses represents an insurance policy against these and other factors that can deplete your food of its nutritional value. Physicians do not always agree on the exact amount of a supplement people should take, but the suggested dosages given below are a general consensus. They can help you choose a multiple vitamin-mineral supplement. Consult with your physician, who may recommend additional levels of some supplements, depending on your activity level and general health.

Beta-carotene	5,000–25,000 IU
Biotin	100–300 mcg
Boron	1–2 mg
Calcium	250–750 mg
Choline	10–100 mg
Chromium	200–400 mcg
Copper	1–2 mg
Folic acid	200–400 mcg
Inositol	10–100 mg
Iodine	50–150 mcg
Iron	15–30 mg
Magnesium	250–500 mg
Manganese	10–15 mg
Molybdenum	10–25 mcg
Niacin	10–100 mg
Niacinamide	10–30 mg

Pantothenic acid	25–100 mg
Potassium	200–500 mg
Selenium	100–200 mcg
Silica	200–1,000 mcg
Vanadium	50–100 mcg
Vitamin A (retinol)	5,000 IU
Vitamin B_1 (thiamine)	10–100 mg
Vitamin B_2	10–100 mg
Vitamin B_6	25–100 mg
Vitamin B_{12}	200–400 mcg
Vitamin C	100–250 mg
Vitamin D	100–400 IU
Vitamin E (d-alpha tocopherol)	400–800 IU
Vitamin K	60–300 mcg
Zinc	15–30 mg

RECOMMENDED DAILY ALLOWANCES

Below are the latest figures for the Recommended Daily Allowances (RDAs) and Estimated Minimum Daily Requirements (EMDRs) of vitamins and minerals for adults. Not all physicians agree on the value of these figures. Some say they are minimum standards and represent the bottom line for preventing deficiency conditions. Others insist they are safe maximum standards. If you eat a well-balanced diet, you should have little or no problem meeting and in some cases exceeding the RDAs. If you believe you need additional intake of any one or more nutrients, consult with your physician before starting a supplement program.

RDAs AND EMDRs FOR VITAMINS AND MINERALS

FAT-SOLUBLE VITAMINS

These vitamins are stored in the body and so do not need to be consumed daily.

Vitamin A	Women: 4,000 IU or 2.4 mg beta-carotene
	Men: 5,000 IU or 3 mg beta-carotene
Vitamin D	Adults: 200 IU or 5 mcg
	Pregnant women: 400 IU or 10 mcg
Vitamin E	Adults: 400 IU
Vitamin K	Women: 65 mcg
	Men: 80 mcg

WATER-SOLUBLE VITAMINS

Any excess amounts of water-soluble vitamins are eliminated through urination. These vitamins should be consumed daily.

Biotin	Adults: 30–100 mcg
Folate	Adults: 400 mcg
Niacin	Women: 15 mg
	Pregnant women: 17 mg
	Men: 19 mg
Pantothenic acid	Adults: 4–7 mg
Vitamin B_1	Women: 1.1 mg
	Men: 1.5 mg
Vitamin B_2	Women: 1.3 mg
	Pregnant women: 1.6 mg
	Men: 1.7 mg
Vitamin B_6	Women: 1.6 mg
	Pregnant women: 2.2 mg
	Men: 2 mg
Vitamin B_{12}	Adults: 2 mcg
	Pregnant women: 2.2 mcg
Vitamin C	Adults: 200–400 mg

MINERALS

| Calcium | Adults: 800–1,000 mg; 1,500 mg after age 65 |

Chloride	EMDR: 750 mg
Chromium	EMDR: 50–200 mcg
Copper	EMDR: 1.5–3 mg
Fluoride	EMDR: 1.5–4 mg
Iron	Adults: 10 mg
	Pregnant women: 0.30 mg
	Premenopausal women: 15mg
Magnesium	Women: 280 mg
	Pregnant women: 320 mg
	Men: 350 mg
Manganese	EMDR: 2.5–5 mg
Molybdenum	EMDR: 75–250 mcg
Phosphorus	Adults over 25: 800 mg
	Young adults and pregnant women: 1,200 mg
Potassium	EMDR: 2,000 mg
Iodine	EMDR: 150 mcg
Selenium	Women: 55 mcg
	Pregnant women: 65 mcg
	Men: 70 mcg
Sodium	EMDR: 500 mcg
Zinc	Adults: 15 mg
	Pregnant women: 30 mg

5. Buyer Beware: What to Know About Buying Broccoli Sprouts and Other Cancer-Fighting Foods

AFTER READING THE FIRST FIVE CHAPTERS, YOU'RE READY TO improve your diet. You're excited about including broccoli sprouts and other cancer-preventive foods in your menu. After looking through the menus and recipes, you've made a list of ingredients you need. So you pick up the newspaper and see the supermarket circulars that advertise "fresh produce," "crisp, fresh lettuce," "firm, ripe tomatoes," and "luscious, juicy berries." Sounds good.

As you walk into your local supermarket and stand in the produce aisle, you notice the signs hanging above the fruits and vegetables that say the produce has been waxed with paraffin or "food grade beeswax." You start to think about what else may be on the vegetables. When Environmental Protection Agency (EPA) spokesman Al Heier was asked about the millions of pounds of pesticides applied to food crops each year, he said, "We don't believe they pose an unreasonable risk." But then you read a report from the National Academy of Sciences that says an estimated twenty thousand cases of cancer are caused by those very same pesticides on your food. Suddenly you're looking at fruits and vegetables with suspicion. Should you be alarmed? How do you know if the broccoli sprouts and other produce and grains you buy are safe to eat? What is the difference between conventionally grown and organically grown produce? What can you do to protect yourself against unseen toxic residues on your food?

In this chapter I discuss the answers to these and other related questions about the safety and nutritional value of the cancer-fighting foods you buy.

PRODUCE: SERVED WITH PESTICIDES

According to the National Resources Defense Council, 845 million pounds of pesticides, herbicides, and fungicides were applied to American crops in 1997. This practice is not confined to the United States. Many foreign countries, including Mexico (which exports food to the United States), continue to use known carcinogenic agents, like DDT, which have been banned in the United States. This method of farming, usually referred to as conventional farming, is all done in the name of protecting crops from disease and insect damage and to eliminate weeds. Many of these substances, which have been designed to kill, have not been adequately tested to determine their effect on human health.

A significant number of the pesticides approved for agricultural use by the EPA were registered before they underwent extensive research to determine their health risks. The result is that the EPA now considers 90 percent of all fungicides, 60 percent of all herbicides, and 30 percent of all insecticides to be carcinogenic. All of these toxins on food are apparently having a big effect. According to a 1987 National Academy of Sciences report, use of pesticides might cause an additional 1.4 million cases of cancer among Americans. In addition to cancer, pesticides are linked to birth defects, nerve damage, and genetic mutation.

One group that exemplifies the toxic effects of these pesticides is farm workers. A National Cancer Institute study found that farmers who are exposed to herbicides have a six-fold greater risk of developing cancer than do nonfarmers. Since 1973, the number of reported pesticide poisonings among farm workers has increased an average of 14 percent a year and doubled between 1975 and 1985.

The most widely used pesticide in the United States today is malathion, an organophosphate that is lethal to both animals and humans. It is applied by crop-dusting planes, over a wide variety of crops. Malathion was introduced and hailed as a replacement for DDT, a known carcinogenic agent that has been banned in the United States since 1972 but is still used extensively around the world. Thus produce shipped to the United States from foreign countries has the potential to be tainted with DDT. Residues of DDT can still be found in the United States both in the environment and in the bodies of many women, as it is associated with the development of breast cancer.

Other pesticides currently in use include endosulfan, dicofol, and methoxychlor. According to the Environmental Working Group, a private organization, more than two million pounds of endosulfan are used on crops in the United States each year, including carrots, lettuce, tomatoes, spinach, and others. All three of these pesticides act as estrogenic agents, which means they have an estrogenlike effect on the body. Thus they, like DDT, have the potential to cause breast cancer.

HOW FRESH IS FRESH? WHERE HAVE THE NUTRIENTS GONE?

As soon as vegetables and fruits are harvested, they begin to lose flavor and nutritional value. If you have a garden and can pick your own vegetables, you know how fresh they are. But chances are that the lettuce, tomatoes, cucumbers, sprouts, onions, and other salad fixings you purchased at your local supermarket were trucked in from perhaps more than two thousand miles away. Unless you know that the produce you buy is from a local grower and that it was picked within perhaps a matter of hours, the fruits and vegetables you ate today were likely transported and stored in a refrigerated truck, then transferred to another refrigeration unit in the store, before being placed on the shelf. It typically takes up to five days for produce to reach the supermarket shelf. In some cases, especially if the product is grown on one coast and must be shipped to the other or if the items are coming from another country, the lag time between harvest and market can be fourteen days and longer.

Somewhere between the time they were harvested and the time they appeared in the produce aisle, it is very likely the fruit and vegetables you are contemplating were chemically treated in some way. Americans like their produce to "look good." To satisfy that desire, as well as lengthen the shelf life of fruits and vegetables, produce handlers often wash their products in chlorinated water to kill bacteria and mold. Fruits and vegetables such as cucumbers, apples, and squash are routinely given a coating of wax or paraffin until they look artificial. This practice slows decay, reduces water loss, and makes the produce look "perfect." Dyes are applied to citrus to make the skins aesthetically pleasing. Sprout inhibitors are applied to potatoes and onions to hinder sprouting during storage.

Generally, fruits and vegetables are cooled very soon after harvest in order to ensure marketability and freshness. A loss of nutritional value is inevitable, however, and the first to fade are the water-soluble vitamins, such as vitamin C and the B vitamins (thiamine, riboflavin, niacin, B_6 and B_{12}). In fact, food and nutrition experts use the decay of vitamin C as an indicator of how many other nutrients have been lost. One example is strawberries. After being stored for two weeks at 41° Fahrenheit (not an unusual length of time), they lose about 20 percent of their vitamin C.

The nutritional value of produce is also compromised when it is picked before it is ripe. Growers are often forced to harvest their crops before they are ripe because the products need to be shipped long distances, and harvesting fully mature fruits and vegetables would result in spoiled product. Studies show that among some varieties of tomatoes, 30 percent of the vitamin C is lost when the tomatoes are picked while still green.

Handling and/or storage of produce also robs it of its nutritional value, especially when poor or improper procedures are followed and produce gets bruised. In addition to vitamins and minerals, many cancer-fighting phytochemicals are lost. Because there are so many phytochemicals, and research in this field is relatively new, scientists have not yet determined how much phytochemical content is affected by storage, processing, and aging. Johns Hopkins University researcher Jed Fahey, who is faculty research associate and manager of the Brassic Chemo Protection Laboratory, has found that isothiocyanates and glucosinolates, two important cancer-fighting phytochemicals found in broccoli and other cruciferous vegetables, lose potency over time.

CREATING SAFE PRODUCE?

While conventionally grown produce is contaminated from the outside, now there is also internal contamination going on. Genetic engineering is a process by which molecular biologists manipulate the genes of fruits, vegetables, grains, and other plants to produce a "better"—and economically more viable—product. High on the list of desirable traits is a slower decay process so produce will have a longer shelf life. To accomplish this, scientists are transferring genes from one species to another: for example, injecting fish and insect genes into vegetables, and bacteria genes into corn.

What effect does genetic manipulation have on the body in general and on nutritional value in particular? According to Laura Tiaciatti, executive director of Mothers for Natural Law, a nonprofit organization that is concerned about the dangers of genetically engineered food, the dangers are unknown. She notes that because "plants are holistic systems in which everything affects everything else," tampering with the genetic makeup could result in potentially serious problems, perhaps even worse than those associated with the use of pesticides. Already there is evidence that such food tampering is triggering allergic reactions in some people who are sensitive to the substance that has been injected into the genetically altered food. As of 1997, genetically modified foods made up 14 percent of products on the market. It is estimated that modified produce will dominate the market within a few years. For more information about genetic engineering, see Appendix A.

DEFINING "ORGANIC"

As of April 1998, only eleven states required specific standards for certifying foods and crops as organic. Among those states, however, there are differences as to what "organic" means, which pesticides are considered toxic, and what constitutes organic agricultural methods. Thus a "certified organic" orange from California may not fit the bill in Georgia, and vice versa.

However, there are general principles organic farmers follow in regard to how they view their connection with nature, deal with insect pests, fertilize the soil, and raise their crops. Their perspectives and practices differ from those of conventional farmers, and those differences have an impact on the taste and nutritional value of the food they grow.

Organic farmers, for example, believe in forming a balanced partnership with nature so natural processes can occur. This means they avoid use of synthetic fertilizers and chemical pesticides, herbicides, and fungicides, which upset the natural balance and place stress on the plants. A stressed plant is not a healthy one, nor does it taste as good as it could.

To organic growers, the soil is the most basic and important factor in the food they produce. For them, soil is a living organism that needs to be fed well and routinely. The "feed" can consist of compost (a mixture of organic materials that are allowed to decay naturally to produce a rich soil), straw, mulch, and naturally derived nutrients such as powdered fish or greensand. A soil rich in nutrients passes along those beneficial ingredients to the plants that grow in it.

Therein lies another major difference between conventional and organic growers. Conventional farmers dump toxins and synthetic compounds on top of and into the soil in attempts to kill weeds and insects. They do not view soil as the first vital step in producing nutritious, living food. As a result, the fruits, vegetables, and grains harvested from this soil are weak or lacking in vital nutrients, as well as carriers of toxic residues.

As for insect and weed control, here again organic growers shun a toxic approach. Insect traps and barriers, row covers (thin, sun-sensitive material that covers the plants but lets the sun in), and treatment with natural insecticides such as mineral oil and certain types of soap are all part of the organic growers' arsenal. Sometimes it is necessary to bring in beneficial insects to do natural battle with the "bad guys." An invasion of aphids, for example, can be fought naturally by releasing ladybugs in the infected area. Ladybugs feed vigorously on aphids.

THE PUSH FOR NATIONAL ORGANIC STANDARDS

In an attempt to establish an industry standard for organic food, the U.S. Department of Agriculture introduced an extensive list of proposed standards in December 1997. The agency had been working on the proposal for eight years, and the proposed guidelines were received, at least initially, with enthusiasm by organic farmers and the public. A more careful inspection of the proposals by consumer groups and organic growers, however, revealed some suggested practices that could undermine existing organic practices. Some of the most controversial proposals include the following:

- possible use of synthetic chemicals banned under current organic standards
- increased use of antibiotics and nonorganic feed for livestock
- failure to establish policy concerning genetically engineered crops, irradiation of food, and the use of sewage sludge to fertilize crops

The organic standards that come out of the hearings to establish federal standards will have a tremendous effect on the quality of produce in this country and ultimately on your health.

When buying produce for you and your family, it is clearly a matter of "buyer beware." You also need to be aware of what can happen to your food before it reaches your plate and your options in assuring you get the best quality and nutrition you can buy.

Organic produce, grains, legumes, seeds, and nuts, while not perfect, are clearly the better health choice. If you use conventionally grown fruits and vegetables, you need to take extra care when preparing them. In either case, the extra attention you take with the food you and your family eats is well worth the added insurance you get against cancer and other diseases.

HOW TO REDUCE YOUR RISK FROM PESTICIDES ON FOOD

• Whenever possible, buy certified organically grown produce and products made with organic grains and legumes. Organic produce is currently grown and harvested under strict guidelines that ensure the fruits and vegetables are free of pesticides, chemicals, and artificial fertilizers. Because organically grown produce has not been treated with preservatives and other chemicals, you know you're getting the freshest produce when you purchase it. That also means you need to use it relatively quickly, before it spoils. Organic produce tends to be more expensive than conventionally grown items, but you'll be getting a healthier, better quality product.

• Shop at farmers' markets. Often you can find organic produce there, or at least produce that is fresher than what is available in the supermarket and that has been treated with a minimal amount of pesticides. To locate a farmers' market in your area, call your local state or county Farm Bureau. You can also contact the USDA Agricultural Marketing Service at 202-720-8317 and ask for a copy of the farmers' market directory. A list of farmers' markets by state is available on the Internet at www.ams.usda.gov/tmd/markets/states.htm

• Try mail order or home delivery services of organic produce. These can be pricey alternatives, and in the case of mail order, not all items are available. (Several mail order sources are listed at the end of this chapter.) Another option is home delivery. Enterprising entrepreneurs in many cities and towns have started home delivery services of organic produce. Typically, for a set price you can get a container of seasonal vegetables and fruits delivered to your home on a predetermined delivery schedule or as needed.

• An option that is growing in popularity is the Community-Supported Agriculture program, or CSA. In this system, individuals join together and contract with one or more local farmers to buy a specific amount of produce. These individuals are shareholders in the CSA, and the money they pay up front guarantees they will receive fresh produce each week during the growing season, delivered to one or more specified locations. Most CSAs provide all or primarily organic food. (To obtain a free copy of CSAs operating in the United States, call the Biodynamic Farming and Gardening Association at 1-800-516-7797, or mail your request to PO Box 550, Kimberton, PA 19442.)

Community-Supported Agriculture programs are a win-win situation for local farmers and consumers. Local, often small or medium-size organic farmers can be guaranteed an outlet and steady income for their products while consumers get fresh, nutritionally sound produce.

• If possible, grow your own fruits and vegetables. You may not even need your own space in which to do it! Some cities and towns have community gardens where people who don't have their own garden space can plant crops and reap their own harvest. Call your local gardening club, agricultural extension office, or organic growers' club to see if community gardens exist in your area.

When you're not able to get organic produce, there are steps you can take to reduce your risk from pesticides and other toxic substances on your food.

- **Wash all fruits and vegetables** in water with a small amount of mild dish detergent, preferably an antibacterial soap, to remove pesticides that are not water soluble. Then rinse them thoroughly with clear water and scrub them with a vegetable brush (available in most department stores and supermarkets). For leafy vegetables like lettuce and spinach, place leaves in a small tub or pot of water, squish well, dump out the water and rinse the leaves again, but do not allow the leaves to soak in the water. Soaking vegetables and fruits can remove nutrients. Wash organically grown produce, as well. There are also commercially available vegetable "washes," such as Vegiwash, sold in health food stores and by mail order.

- **Peel fruits and vegetables** and remove the outer leaves from lettuce, cabbage, and brussels sprouts. Unfortunately, this removes some of the nutrients and much of the fiber. You do not need to peel organic produce.

- **Beware of fruits and vegetables that have a shiny coating.** They have been waxed with paraffin, which may or may not be carcinogenic. If you do buy waxed fruits and vegetables, definitely peel them before eating.

- **Eat a variety of fruits and vegetables.** This will lessen your exposure to high concentrations of pesticides on one food.

- **Ask your supermarket to carry organically grown produce.**

- **Support local farmers who grow organic produce.**

BUYING BROCCOLI SPROUTS

Broccoli sprouts are literally "sprouting up" all over the country in health food stores, food cooperatives, mainstream supermarkets, natural food stores, farmers' markets, and roadside stands. If they have not made their way to your area, encourage your local produce managers to get them. Also, check your local telephone directory or classified advertising section under "Produce" or "Farm Products" to see if you have a produce delivery service in your town. This is becoming a popular business across the nation. In the meantime, you can order broccoli sprouts and other organically grown produce through the mail.

MAIL ORDER SOURCES OF ORGANIC PRODUCTS

Cascadian Farm
Sedro-Woolley, WA
303-403-4022

Diamond Organics
Freedom, CA 95019
800-922-2396

GoodEats
PO Box 756
Richboro, PA 18954
800-490-0044
www.goodeats.com/

Grass Roots
PO Box 77893
Tucson, AZ 85703
520-623-7240

Starr Organic Produce
PO Box 561502
Miami, FL 33256
305-262-1242

Walnut Acres Organic Farms
Penns Creek, PA 17862
800-433-3998

World Variety Produce (Melissa's)
5325 S. Soto Street
Vernon, CA 90058
800-588-0151

6. When in Doubt, Grow Your Own

THERE'S SOMETHING VERY REWARDING AND SATISFYING ABOUT growing your own food. From the time you prepare the soil and plant the seeds, until you reap the fruits of your toils, you can share in the wonder of growth.

You don't need a yard or a lot of space to grow your own vegetables. If you have a few strategically placed pots in the house or on the porch, or if you have hanging plants, window boxes, or trays under a grow lamp in a corner of your garage, you can yield an adequate supply of fresh produce.

Growing sprouts is even easier than other vegetables. When you grow sprouts, you embark on a new type of "farming" experience. Forget the hoes and rakes; you'll be using glass jars, rubber bands, and cheesecloth. There are no weeds to pick and no bugs to chase away. Best of all, you can reap your harvest within days, instead of months. And your crop will be rich in vitamins, minerals, and protein.

This chapter explains how you can become a sprout farmer in your own kitchen. Included are instructions on how to grow broccoli sprouts and other nutritious sprouts and where to get the best seeds for sprouting. After a few days, you'll be ready to try your harvest in the recipes presented in Chapter 7.

GETTING STARTED

Sprouting does not require any fancy equipment, but you do need to start with quality seed. Look for a reputable seed supplier, like those listed at the end of this chapter. You want to use *untreated* sprouting seed. This differs from seed destined for planting in the soil, which is often treated with fungicides to prevent rotting or decay. When you receive the seed, immediately store it in a sealed container and put it in a dry, dark place until you are ready to sprout it. Optimal storage temperature for seed is between 65° and 75° F.

You'll need a very fine sieve so you can rinse the seed. Make sure the mesh is tight enough to prevent the tiny broccoli seeds from falling through. Alfalfa seeds also are very small. Sieves can be purchased in the kitchen gadget section of department stores. You have your choice of sprouting methods: jar, flowerpot, plate, or commercial sprouting kit:

- Jar: Mason-type jars are a favorite, although any wide-mouth jar is sufficient. You will need a piece of cheesecloth, fine muslin, or fine screen to place over the opening. Secure the material with a rubber band or string.

- Flowerpot: Select a plastic flowerpot and cheesecloth, muslin, or fine screen to cover the top. A clay pot can be used; however, see precautions mentioned below.

- Plate: Choose a large ceramic or stainless steel platter, preferably a serving-size platter with a lip. You will also need cling wrap to cover the plate.

- Sprouting kit: There are several different styles of sprouting kits. Some consist of several tiers, which allow the water to drain to the bottom tier. Tiered sprouters also let you watch the growing process. Others include glass jars or tubes with various appropriate mesh lids that allow you to sprout seeds of different sizes.

SPROUTING BROCCOLI SEEDS

The following instructions are for the jar method; guidelines for the other approaches follow.

Jar Method

1. Place 2 tablespoons of seeds on a fine-mesh sieve and rinse under running water.

2. Place the rinsed seeds in the sprouting jar and add four times as much lukewarm water as seeds (about 8 tablespoons of water). Secure the cover over the jar opening and allow the seeds to soak for about twelve hours.

3. Pour out the water the seeds soaked in. Rinse the seeds again by adding water to the jar and pouring it out.

4. Position the jar at a slight angle, mesh-covered opening down, over a cup or other container so excess water can drain off. Place the jar in a dark closet or cupboard.

5. Rinse the seeds two or three times a day. Hold the covered jar under slowly running water and allow the jar to overflow. Invert the jar and let the water drain out. When rinsing, do not shake the bottle—the developing sprouts are very fragile. Rinsing helps remove the tough hulls from the sprouts.

6. After three or four days, the sprouts will be ready for their final touch—chlorophyll. Place the jar on a windowsill for a few hours of indirect sunlight (direct sunlight will dry them out) or under a lamp. The tiny leaves of the sprouts will turn green as they create chlorophyll.

• An alternative method is to leave the jar at an angle in light, but not direct sunlight, instead of a dark closet or cupboard. Rinse as directed above. After three to four days, the sprout leaves should appear, and the sprouts will be ready for eating.

Flowerpot Method

1. Choose either a clay or plastic flowerpot that has drainage holes in the bottom. If clay, clean it thoroughly and let the pot sit in clean water for a few hours and absorb the water. This is important, because an "untreated" clay pot draws water away from the sprouts, and they will dry out and die.

2. Follow steps 1 through 3 under Jar Method above, using the flowerpot instead of a jar.

3. Place a piece of fine-mesh netting in the bottom of the pot and put the rinsed seeds into the pot. Cover the top of the flowerpot with a plate.

4. Rinse the seeds two to three times a day by placing the flowerpot under a light-spray faucet.

5. Follow step 6 above.

Platter Method

This method is recommended for sprouting seeds and beans that develop a jellylike coating when they sprout; for example, mustard seed, radish seed, and common cress. This method is not recommended for broccoli sprouts.

1. Follow step 1 under Jar Method above.

2. Spread the seeds out evenly on the platter and add 2 tablespoons of water to the platter. After a few hours, check the water level. The seeds should be wet but not floating.

3. Cover the seeds with a sheet of cling wrap into which you have punched a few small holes. Place the platter in a dark place.

4. Use a spray bottle to wet the seeds two to four times a day. The sprouts will be ready in about four days.

5. Follow step 6 above.

Sprouting Hints

- Soak seeds in warm water, rinse them in tepid water, and do the final rinse of the sprouts in cold water.

- The soaking water is full of nutrients. Use it to make soup broth or to water your plants.

- To reduce problems with moldy seeds or sprouts, remove the hulls during the rinsing process. Dehulled sprouts tend to be tastier; however, some people like the hulls because they add fiber. If you keep the hulls on, watch for mold.

- If the sprouts begin to get moldy, sour, or dried out, throw them away or add them to your compost pile. Soybean sprouts are the most likely ones to become sour if they are not rinsed regularly enough.

- Most sprouts will remain fresh in the refrigerator for three to five days, or up to 10 days if stored in a tight container. If you have an abundance of sprouts and need to use them quickly, make one of the delicious recipes in Chapter 7.

- Some people say never freeze sprouts; others say it's okay. If you do freeze them, parboil them first to avoid them going sour.

- Do not let your sprouts grow too long. If the recommended growing time is three days, harvest them then. Sprouts that are allowed to grow too long can become bitter and stale and lose their crunchy texture.

- If you do let a batch get too long but they are not bitter, don't despair. Instead of eating them raw, use them in a recipe that requires cooking.

- If there is not adequate sunlight to "green" your sprouts, place them in a room with electric light.

- To speed up the greening process, spread out the sprouts on a tray before placing them in the light.

- Refrigerate sprouts immediately after they are green. This allows the life force to stay in the seed and continue to gain in nutritional value. If they are left out at room temperature after harvest, the vitamins and other nutrients will start to decompose.

SPROUTING OUT

Along with broccoli sprouts, you may want to try some of the many other sprouts. Though broccoli sprouts are an important addition to a healthful, cancer-prevention eating plan, the addition of other sprouts to your menu can add essential nutrients, as well as variety. Here is information on a few other sprouts you can grow on your own (or in some cases, purchase ready to eat):

- *Alfalfa.* This tiny seed yields what many call the "king of the sprouts." Alfalfa sprouts contain as much carotene as carrots and are the sprout highest in levels of protein, minerals, and vitamins A, B complex, C, D, E, and K. Soak the seeds for six to twelve hours and harvest in three to seven days, depending on the size of sprouts you desire. Alfalfa sprouts should be harvested before the leaves appear, however, to derive the greatest nutritional value. Use a bottle, sprouter, or tube to sprout these tiny seeds.

- *Buckwheat.* Buckwheat contains all of the essential amino acids. Purchase unhulled buckwheat for sprouting. After rinsing the seeds initially, do not soak them. Do rinse them three to four times a day, however. They should be ready to eat in two to three days. Use a bottle or tube for sprouting.

- *Cabbage.* Cabbage sprouts are rich in minerals and the antioxidant vitamins A and C. Start with 1/3 cup seeds and soak them for four to six hours. Cabbage seeds take four to five days to sprout. After harvesting, rinse them thoroughly to remove the hulls. Use a bottle or tube for sprouting.

- *Corn.* Corn sprouts are a good source of vitamin A and potassium. The soaking time on these seeds is twelve hours, but they sprout in only two to three days. Start with 1 cup of sweet corn seeds. You will need to remove the hulls after harvesting. Use a bottle or flowerpot method for sprouting.

• *Fenugreek.* This unique tasting sprout is rich in vitamin A and protein. These sprouts are ready to eat after three days, but wait until the leaves have developed, which occurs by day five. Don't delay, however, because they can become bitter if the sprout grows too long. Use a bottle, flowerpot, or tube to sprout.

• *Lentils.* The sprouts of this legume are high in the antioxidant vitamins A, C, and E and are a complete protein. Lentils are easy to sprout if their hulls are intact. Soak them for twelve hours and then rinse them two to four times a day. They are ready to eat after three to four days. Use any sprouting method for these seeds.

• *Millet.* These sprouts are rich in protein, phosphorus, iron, calcium, riboflavin, and niacin. After rinsing the seeds, soak them for six to twelve hours. Rinse the seeds two to four times a day. Millet will sprout in three to four days and is ready to eat when the sprout is the same length as the seed. Use the bottle or sprouter.

• *Mung Beans.* Perhaps the best-known sprout is that of the mung bean, which is found in traditional Chinese food. Mung bean sprouts are high in calcium, vitamins A and C, protein, phosphorus, and iron. Soak the seeds for twelve hours, then rinse two to three times daily. Wait until the sprouts have two tiny leaves before eating them. Use any sprouting method for these seeds.

• *Peas.* Pea sprouts contain all the essential amino acids, as well as vitamins A, B_1, and C. Soak the peas for twelve hours, then rinse them three times a day. The sprouts are ready in three days; too much longer and they will become tough. Use the bottle or tube method to sprout.

• *Radish and Mustard Seed.* The sprouts of both radish and mustard have a strong, "bitey" taste. Use the platter method or a sprouter for these sprouts. After you rinse the seeds, do not soak them. Rinse or spray them with a mist two to four times a day, and they will be ready in three to four days.

• *Soybeans.* Soybean sprouts have a very high protein content (40 percent) and are rich in vitamins B and C. These sprouts are a bit more challenging to grow than other sprouting seeds, yet their nutritional value is worth the effort. Soak the beans for about twelve hours, then rinse them four to six times a day. In three to five days you can harvest. Use a bottle, flowerpot, or tube to sprout.

• *Wheat.* Wheat sprouts are a good source of protein, calcium, iron, and vitamins B, C, and E. Sprouting wheat is easy, as is sprouting barley, oats, and rye. Soaking time is twelve hours, then rinse the wheat two to three times a day. After a short growing time (three to four days), you'll be ready to enjoy wheat sprouts. Use any sprouting method for these seeds.

WHY SPROUT?

Sprouts are one of the most nutritional and complete foods you can eat. You already know that broccoli sprouts contain up to one hundred times the amount of sulforaphane found in mature broccoli. But this powerful antioxidant is not the only nutrient that appears in significantly higher levels in broccoli sprouts: Vitamins A and C, and various other phytochemicals also appear in greater amounts in the sprouts. And these enhanced levels hold true for other sprouts as well.

Sprouts are living food because they contain living cells, unlike food that is processed or cooked. During the sprouting process, the seed undergoes powerful chemical changes that dramatically increase the levels of various nutrients. In wheat, for example, levels of vitamin B_{12} increase fourfold, while other B vitamins increase three to twelve times, and vitamin E increases threefold. The amount of vitamin A in mung bean sprouts is more than twice that in the dry bean. In some cases, a nutrient appears in the sprout that is not found in the mature plant. Dry beans, seeds, and legumes, for example, do not contain vitamin C. But when you sprout them, a 3½-ounce serving contains about 20 milligrams.

A unique feature of sprouts is that even after you harvest them and put them in the refrigerator, their nutritional value increases, because they are living foods. This is in sharp contrast with all other fruits and vegetables.

Growing your own sprouts gives you powerful, anticancer nutrition at your fingertips, anytime of the year. When the snow is piled up at your doorstep, you'll have a fresh source of highly nutritious vegetables in the warmth of your kitchen.

Another advantage to growing your own sprouts is that you can refrigerate them immediately after harvest, which preserves the ability of the sprouts to continue to grow in nutritional value. Sprouts bought in the market have begun to lose vitamins and other nutrients because they have been left out at room temperature. By the time you get them home and refrigerated, they have lost some of their nutrients.

Sprouting seeds makes it very easy for the body to digest them, because sprouting breaks protein down into amino acids and concentrated starch into simple carbohydrates. Sprouts also provide an abundance of special enzymes that help the body's digestive process. These enzymes are found only in raw foods, and sprouted seeds, grains, and legumes are the best source of these enzymes.

WHERE TO GET BROCCOLI AND OTHER SPROUTING SEEDS

The following companies carry untreated sprouting seeds; some also carry sprouting kits. Several of these companies can be contacted via the Internet to place orders, request a catalog, ask questions, and view other products.

W. Atlee Burpee & Company
300 Park Avenue
Warminster, PA 18974
800-888-1447; customer service 1-800-333-5808
http://garden.burpee.com/
Free catalog available.
Mariner hybrid is a potent variety of broccoli sprouts.
Available in any size seed package and in seed strips.

Edrich Farms
410-922-5700
Sprouting seeds

Greenheart Farms
Box 1510
Arroyo Grande, CA 93421
805-481-2234
Sprouting seeds

Johnny's Selected Seeds
Foss Hill Road
Albion, ME 04910-9731
207-437-4301
www.johnnyseeds.com/
Free catalog available; has seed sprouters.

Piedmont Plant Co.
PO Box 424
Albany, GA 31702
912-883-7029
Ask for free catalog.

Pinetree Garden Seed
616A Lewiston Road
New Gloucester, ME 04260
207-926-3400
www.superseeds.com/
Sprouting seeds

Seeds of Change
PO Box 15700
Santa Fe, NM 87506
1-888-762-7333
Sprouting seeds

The Sprout House
17267 Sundance Drive
Ramona, CA 92065
1-800-777-6887 (1-800-SPROUTS)
Sprouting seeds available in quantities of ¼ pound and up.

The Sproutpeople
225 Main Street
Gays Mills, WI 54631
608-735-4735
www.sproutpeople.com/broccoli.html
Sprouting seeds

Territorial Seed Co.
PO Box 157
Cottage Grove, OR 97424
541-942-9547
Sprouting seeds

Shepherd's Garden Seeds
30 Irene Street
Torrington, CT 06790
203-482-3638
www.shepherdseeds.com/
Ask for free catalog.

Walton Feed, Inc.
135 North 10th
PO Box 307
Montpelier, ID 83254
800-269-8563
Sprouting seeds

Also check your local health food stores, organic gardening association, organic farm groups, and county agricultural extension offices for sprouting seeds and sprouting
containers.

7. Your Cancer-Prevention Eating Program: Two Weeks of Menus and Recipes

THE TIME HAS COME TO TAKE ALL THE INFORMATION YOU'VE read so far and put it to practical use. You're ready to add broccoli sprouts to your menu, but you don't know what to do with them. You've seen the list of cancer-fighting foods, but you're feeling a bit overwhelmed when you think about how to incorporate them into your daily eating plans. This chapter brings it all together for you: two weeks of cancer-fighting recipes and menu ideas, presented day-by-day.

INCORPORATING BROCCOLI SPROUTS INTO YOUR DIET

To help you add broccoli sprouts to your daily diet, they have been included as a part of the menu plans below, and each recipe with sprouts as an ingredient is marked with ✓. Generally, experts believe that in terms of cancer protection, about 1 ounce of broccoli sprouts is equal to 2 pounds of mature broccoli. One ounce of broccoli sprouts equals approximately 30 grams; 30 grams equals approximately 1 cup of lightly packed broccoli sprouts; and 1 ounce of sprouts per week is the amount experts believe to be adequate to reduce the risk of cancer by as much as 50 percent for some cancers, such as colon cancer. Of course, you are welcome to eat more!

The recipes and menus in this chapter contain the recommended amount of broccoli sprouts for cancer protection. If you would like to experiment on your own with broccoli sprouts, here are some ways you can use them:

- Top your sandwiches and salads with sprouts.
- Add a handful the next time you make vegetable juice in your juicer.
- Add 2–3 tablespoons of chopped sprouts to your home-made bread recipe.
- Add sprouts to any stir-fry about one minute before you are done cooking.
- Add 1 cup of lightly packed sprouts to homemade soup about five minutes before it is ready.
- Chop sprouts and sauté them with onion in any recipe that calls for sautéed onion, peppers, mushrooms, etc.
- Spread a layer of sprouts under the sauce of a home-made pizza.
- Sprinkle a layer of sprouts on a bean burrito before rolling it up.
- Add a layer of sprouts to lasagna.
- Add 1 to 2 cups (lightly packed) sprouts to any stuffing recipe.
- Finely chop sprouts and add to dips or sandwich spreads, like the Eye-Opening Eggplant or Great Garbanzo spreads in the recipes below.

HOW TO USE THE RECIPES AND MENU IDEAS

Every person who picks up this book has different dietary habits and food preferences, as well as different ways he or she makes changes in eating patterns. So where possible and nutritionally sound, I offer optional ingredients so you can choose which item you want to try. Giving you this choice is good for several reasons:

- It allows you to substitute for ingredients you do not have on hand or don't have readily available.

- Because some of these foods may be very new to you, it lets you make gradual changes to your diet.

- It makes the recipes easy to use for people who already eat a plant-based diet, as well as those who want to make a transition or those who are not ready to change. For example, recipes calling for milk have the option of soy milk, rice milk, or nonfat cow's milk. The Billion Bean Chili recipe offers the option of using tofu or plant-based burgers.

HEALTHFUL EATING MADE EASY

Forget anything you've heard that says healthful eating is boring and tasteless. It's really quite the contrary! The secret is in your perspective. You are *adding* new foods, not giving foods up. You can *modify* your favorite recipes, not stop enjoying them. You will discover new flavors, new textures, and new food combinations. Here are some tips:

- Get a Crock-Pot or slow cooker. These two kitchen appliances are invaluable for making beans, rice, grains, soups, and many one-pot meals.

- Keep your meals simple. (I have kept this in mind and provided easy recipes.) Plan one basic, hearty entrée and add other simple foods around it. You're probably too busy to spend all your time in the kitchen, anyway.

- When making basic foods, such as beans, rice, lentils, split peas, and various grains, make large portions and freeze the excess in small containers to use for later meals. Do the same for one-pot meals, such as chili and stews, and freeze portions to use for a quick lunch or dinner.

- Experiment. Once you've tried a recipe, you may want to make changes that suit your particular taste preferences (choosing healthful substitutions, of course!). This is especially true for herbs and spices. If a recipe calls for fennel and you don't like it, don't toss the recipe; just don't use the fennel, or substitute something you do like.

- Experiment more. Have a favorite soup recipe but want to try something different? Make it with less liquid next time, or thicken the broth and serve the "soup" over toasted whole-grain bread, like a sloppy joe, or over pasta, rice, or other whole grains.

- Pita pockets are an incredibly convenient food. You can stuff just about anything in them, including leftover casseroles and stews, dips, vegetables, and even assorted sliced and mashed fruits.

- Use the water left over from steamed vegetables or from cooking beans to make soup stock. It's loaded with nutrients.

- Use water instead of oil to sauté foods, and use vegetable broth or stock, instead of beef or chicken, in recipes that call for broth.

- Don't use the salt shaker. Try fresh herbs, lemon juice, fresh ground pepper, fresh salsa, and those great cancer fighters onion, garlic, leeks, and chives for flavoring.

MAKING THE TRANSITION TO A PLANT-BASED DIET

If you are not already eating a plant-based diet and want to make some healthful changes, I can help you make the transition easily and with great-tasting recipes. Everyone makes changes at a different pace. If you're not ready to make a complete switch to plant-based eating, begin by reducing the amount of meat, poultry, and dairy products you eat at each meal and the number of times per week that you include them in your diet. Think of these foods as condiments, as people in many cultures do, and use them as such: a few ounces of slivered chicken in a vegetable casserole or stir-fry; a 3- to 4-ounce piece of salmon or other cold-water fish to complement Corny Couscous or Split Pea and Vegetable Stew, for example.

The wide variety of soy- and vegetable-based meat and dairy substitutes available in many supermarkets and health food stores have made the transition to a healthful, plant-based diet convenient and easy for tens of thousands of people. Be willing to experiment. These meat and dairy substitutes have the look, taste, and texture of chicken, beef, and other items they are intended to replace, and without the high fat, cholesterol, hormones, and other food additives found in animal products.

TWO WEEKS OF DAILY MENUS

✓ lets you know that a recipe has been provided. The recipes follow each day's menu.

✗ means that the recipe or menu item includes broccoli sprouts.

A note on the Sandwich Spreads: Use any of the sandwich spreads in whole-wheat pita bread or on whole-wheat or whole-grain rolls or toasted bread. Serve with broccoli sprouts, sliced tomato and cucumber, onion slices, lettuce, or any other favorite sandwich topping. These spreads can double as dips. Just add a few drops of water to the eggplant spread, or a few drops of soy milk to the bean spreads, until they reach the desired consistency.

Day 1

BREAKFAST
    ½ grapefruit
    Apple Pancakes✓
    Herbal tea

LUNCH
   Quick Curried Lentil Soup✓
   Rye crackers
   ✗ Tossed green salad with broccoli sprouts, tomato, pep-
       pers, and fresh-squeezed lemon and chopped chives
       dressing
   Iced herbal tea

DINNER
   Festive Fettuccine✓
   ✗A&C-Burst Coleslaw✓
   1 slice whole-grain bread
   Coffee substitute

SNACK
   Fruit Smoothie✓ (see Smoothie recipes at end of menus,
       page 131)

Apple Pancakes (makes 6–7 pancakes)

   1 cup whole-wheat flour
   ½ cup unsweetened applesauce
   1 teaspoon egg substitute mixed with 2 tablespoons
       water
   1 teaspoon baking powder
   1 cup apple juice
   1 cup grated fresh apple, for topping

*Mix dry ingredients together in a bowl. In another bowl, mix
egg substitute with water. Add applesauce and apple juice.
Add the liquid mixture to the dry ingredients and stir. Pour
batter onto a preheated nonstick griddle or pan and cook
over medium heat. Turn the pancakes when bubbles appear
on the surface. Serve with grated apple.*

Quick Curried Lentil Soup (serves 4)

   5 cups water
   1 cup uncooked lentils

⅓ cup uncooked barley
1 chopped onion
2 teaspoons curry powder
2 small potatoes, diced
1 teaspoon cumin

Combine all ingredients in a soup pot and cook over medium low heat for about 1 hour. (If using a Crock-Pot or slow cooker, cook for 4 hours on high or 8 hours on low.)

Festive Fettuccini (serves 4)

10 ounces fettuccini
2 cloves garlic, minced
½ pound cubed firm tofu, or 1 cup shredded cooked chicken breast
1 tablespoon olive oil
1½ pounds ripe tomatoes, cut into 1-inch pieces
1 cup (packed) fresh basil leaves, slivered
¼ teaspoon ground black pepper
¼ pound asparagus, cut into one-inch pieces
6 brussels sprouts, cut into quarters and steamed
Salt to taste

Cook fettuccini according to package directions. Drain and reserve ⅓ cup cooking liquid. In a large skillet, sauté garlic and tofu in oil for about 1 minute. Add tomatoes and brussels sprouts and reserved liquid. Cook for about 1 minute. Add the pasta (and optional chicken) and toss. Remove from heat and add the basil, salt, and pepper. Serve immediately.

✗A&C-Burst Coleslaw (serves 4)

Called A&C because it is rich in vitamins A and C.

2 cups shredded green cabbage
2 carrots, grated (1 cup)
1 red bell pepper, seeded and slivered
1 papaya, peeled, seeded, and slivered
1 cup (lightly packed) broccoli sprouts

1 clove garlic, minced
¼ cup soy mayonnaise
⅓ cup packed cilantro leaves, chopped
2 tablespoons lemon juice
¼ teaspoon ground black pepper

Combine cabbage, carrots, red pepper, papaya, and sprouts in a bowl. In another bowl, combine garlic, mayonnaise, cilantro, lemon juice, and black pepper. Mix well and add to cabbage mixture. Toss and serve.

Day 2

BREAKFAST
¼ cantaloupe
Nonfat soy yogurt (or nonfat regular yogurt)
Mighty Muffin✓
Decaf tea

LUNCH
✗ Chilled Couscous with Lentils✓ in ½ whole-grain pita
or whole-wheat tortilla wrap with broccoli sprouts
Steamed brussels sprouts with lemon and cilantro
Flavored seltzer

DINNER
Zest of Life Stew✓
Whole-grain roll
Pear Rice Pudding with Kiwi Sauce✓
Vegetable juice

SNACK
Raw vegetable slices (zucchini, carrots, radishes, peppers) with Eye-Opening Eggplant Dip✓

Mighty Muffins (makes 12 muffins)

2 cups whole-wheat flour
2 teaspoons baking powder

½ cup raisins or chopped dried apricots
¼ cup honey
1½ cups soy milk, rice milk, or nonfat milk
2 tablespoons applesauce
1 teaspoon egg substitute mixed with 2 tablespoons
   water

Preheat oven to 350°. Combine the dry ingredients in one bowl and the wet ingredients in another. Fold the dry and wet ingredients together until moist. Spoon the batter into nonstick muffin tins or paper muffin cups. Bake for 30 minutes. Muffins are done when a toothpick inserted into the top center comes out clean.

Chilled Couscous with Lentils (serves 2–4)

½ cup dry lentils
2 cups water
⅓ cup uncooked couscous
½ cup boiling water
½ cup corn kernels
1 small chopped onion
1 tablespoon vegetable oil
1 tablespoon minced cilantro
1 teaspoon red wine vinegar
Salt and pepper to taste

Cook lentils in 2 cups water until tender, about 45 minutes. Drain. Combine couscous and boiling water in a small bowl, cover, and let stand for 5 to 10 minutes. Mix lentils, couscous, and all remaining ingredients. Chill 1 hour before serving.

Zest of Life Stew (serves 6)

2 onions, sliced
2 celery stalks, sliced
½ pound brussels sprouts, halved
½ pound mushrooms, halved

3 large cloves garlic, crushed
3 potatoes, scrubbed and cut into chunks
2 cups water
¼ cup apple juice
¼ cup low-sodium tamari
½ tablespoon grated fresh ginger
½ teaspoon thyme
3–4 tablespoons arrowroot or cornstarch

Combine all ingredients except the arrowroot or cornstarch in a large pot. Bring to a boil, lower heat, cover, and simmer for 90 minutes or until vegetables are tender. Mix the arrowroot in ½ cup water and add the mixture slowly to the stew, stirring constantly until thickened. (In a slow cooker, cook on low for 10 hours or on high for 6 hours.)

Pear Rice Pudding with Kiwi Sauce *(makes 6 cups)*

Also can be served for breakfast.

1 cup uncooked brown rice
2 cups soy milk
1 large apple, peeled and cut in ½-inch dices
4 pears, peeled and cut in ½-inch dices
¼ cup water
4 tablespoons honey or maple syrup
1 teaspoon vanilla extract
⅛ teaspoon ground cinnamon
1 pound kiwi, peeled and chopped
1 teaspoon sugar

In medium saucepan, combine rice and soy milk. Bring to a boil, then reduce heat and simmer for 1 hour. Set aside. Meantime, in another pan, combine apple, pears, water, honey/syrup, vanilla, and cinnamon. Bring to a boil, reduce heat, and simmer for 10 minutes. In a food processor bowl or blender, combine the kiwi and sugar. Puree until smooth. Strain to remove the seeds if desired. Combine the rice and fruit mixtures thoroughly. Serve warm with the kiwi sauce.

Eye-Opening Eggplant Dip (makes 1–1¼ cups)

    1 large eggplant
    2 cloves garlic, minced
    1 green onion, chopped
    ¼ cup chopped parsley
    1 tablespoon lemon juice
    ½ teaspoon dill weed
    10 black olives, pitted

Peel the eggplant and cut it into quarters. Place the pieces into a steam basket and steam until tender, 10 to 15 minutes. When cool, press the liquid out of the eggplant. Place the cooked eggplant and all remaining ingredients except the olives into a blender and blend until smooth. Cut the olives into slivers and add to the eggplant mixture. Chill before using.

Day 3

BREAKFAST
    Southern Comfort Cornmeal with Currants✓
    Soy sausage links
    ½ grapefruit
    Decaf tea

LUNCH
    Almond or peanut butter, all-fruit jelly, and banana on
        whole-grain bread or rolled up in a wheat tortilla
    Tropical fruit mix (guava, pineapple, mango, banana,
        papaya, or whatever is in season)
    Iced herbal tea

DINNER
    ✗Sweet "P" Curry✓
    Brown rice (with optional 3 ounces of broiled chicken
        breast)
    Black-Eyed Beauties✓
    Tomato juice

SNACK
Mighty Muffin✓ (recipe in Day 2)

Southern Comfort Cornmeal with Currants (serves 4)

    4 cups water
    ¾ cup currants
    ¼ teaspoon salt
    1 cup yellow cornmeal
    ½ cup chopped nuts
    ¼ cup sunflower seeds, toasted (optional)

Place water, currants, salt, and cornmeal in a saucepan and bring to a boil, stirring frequently. When it boils, immediately reduce heat to low and simmer, stirring often, for 3 to 5 minutes. Spoon into serving bowls and sprinkle with nuts and sunflower seeds. Serve with rice milk, maple syrup, and cinnamon if desired.

✗Sweet "P" Curry (4–6 servings)

Serve this curry over brown rice, couscous, or barley. Leftovers can be used in pita bread for a spicy sandwich.

    2 onions, sliced
    6 cloves garlic, minced
    2 jalapeño chilies, minced
    1 tablespoon each mustard seed, grated gingerroot, and
      curry powder
    ¼ cup vegetable bouillon
    ½ pound sweet potatoes, peeled and chopped
    ½ pound parsnips, peeled and chopped
    1 28-ounce can plum tomatoes
    Juice of 2 lemons
    1 cup (lightly packed) broccoli sprouts

In a large pot, bring onions, garlic, chilies, spices and bouillon to a boil and simmer 5 to 10 minutes. Add sweet potatoes, parsnips, tomatoes, and lemon juice; cover and simmer

10 minutes. Add broccoli sprouts and simmer for another 5 minutes.

Black-Eyed Beauties

1 cup chopped onion
1 clove garlic, minced
½ cup chopped mushrooms
¼ cup water
1 cup chopped tomatoes (fresh or canned)
3 cups cooked black-eyed peas
1 tablespoon fresh basil, chopped
Salt and pepper to taste

In a large skillet, sauté the onion, garlic, and mushrooms in water until soft. Add the tomatoes and simmer for 1 minute. Add the remaining ingredients and cook for 3 to 4 minutes, stirring gently. Season with salt and pepper to taste.

Day 4

BREAKFAST
Whole-grain fortified cereal with soy or rice milk (or nonfat milk)
Mixed fresh fruit (apple slices, banana, strawberries, grapes, orange sections, cantaloupe, honeydew, as available)
Whole-grain bagel with margarine
Hot decaf tea

LUNCH
✗Sprouted Pizza✓
✗Seaworthy Salad✓ with Herb Dressing✓
Herbal tea

DINNER
Nutty Roast Loaf✓ (or optional 3 ounces broiled mackerel)
Mushroom Gravy✓

Love a Lima Bean Medley✓
Baked potato
Coffee substitute

SNACK
Handful each of dry-roasted nuts and raisins and/or
dried fruit

✗Sprouted Pizza

1 ready-made pizza dough

Preheat the oven to 475° F, or according to package directions. On pizza dough, add toppings of your choice: broccoli sprouts, sliced mushrooms, sliced onion, crushed tomatoes, chopped peppers, shredded nonfat cheese, nutritional yeast, oregano, minced garlic, zucchini slices, black olives.

Suggestion: Spread crushed tomatoes on the dough, top with broccoli sprouts, mushrooms, onion, nutritional yeast, shredded cheese, and more tomatoes. Bake for 10–15 minutes. Serve hot.

Seaworthy Salad (serves 4)

2 cups dried wakame
1 cup dried arame

Soak the wakame and arame in water for about 5 minutes. Drain and cut the wakame into strips, removing the center stem. Place the sea vegetables in a bowl and toss with enough Herb Dressing to suit your taste. Cover and chill about 1 hour before serving.

✗Herb Dressing (makes 1 cup)

½ cup olive oil
¼ cup lemon juice
¼ cup water
¼ cup finely chopped broccoli sprouts

1 clove garlic, crushed
½ teaspoon each parsley, oregano, dill, basil

Mix together the oil, lemon juice, and water. Add the remaining ingredients and shake well.

Nutty Roast Loaf (serves 6–8)

Spray-on cooking oil
1 small onion, chopped
1 stalk celery, chopped
3 cloves garlic, minced
1 tablespoon olive oil (optional)
⅓ cup chopped walnuts
½ cup rolled oats
¼ pound shiitake mushrooms, sliced thin
2 cups water
3 tablespoons each Dijon-style mustard and mild salsa
1 tablespoon soy sauce
1 pound firm tofu, press out water and crumble
3 tablespoons arrowroot
1–1½ cups whole-wheat bread crumbs

Preheat oven to 350°. Lightly spray an 8-cup loaf pan with a spray-on oil. In a skillet, sauté onion, celery, and garlic in oil or a bit of water over medium heat, about 5 minutes. Remove mixture to a small bowl and place walnuts in the skillet and heat about 3 minutes. Stir in oats and mushrooms and sauté over medium heat until the mushrooms get soft (about 5 minutes). Pour in water, raise heat, and simmer for 5 to 10 minutes to reduce liquid. Stir in mustard, salsa, and soy sauce. Continue to cook until the mixture thickens, then add it to the onion mixture. Stir in tofu, arrowroot, and enough bread crumbs to make a firm mixture. Place the mixture into the loaf pan and sprinkle the top with bread crumbs. Bake 40 minutes or until loaf is firm and crust is brown. Cool for 1 hour before slicing.

Mushroom Gravy (makes 2 cups)

1 tablespoon olive oil
2 cups chopped mushrooms
1 small red onion, minced
Salt and pepper to taste
2 cloves garlic, minced
1 tablespoon flour
1 cup soy milk
1 tablespoon nutritional yeast

In a saucepan, heat oil over medium heat. Add mushrooms, onion, garlic, and salt and pepper. Stir often until mushrooms are tender. Reduce heat to low; add flour and nutritional yeast and stir constantly for 1 minute. Add soy milk slowly and continue to stir until the mixture thickens, about 3 minutes.

✗*Love a Lima Bean Medley (serves 2–4)*

2 cloves garlic, minced
2 stalks celery, sliced
2 medium potatoes, diced
1 green pepper, chopped
1 teaspoon dried thyme
1 teaspoon dried marjoram
1 teaspoon olive oil
2 cups water
2 cups corn kernels
1 cup (lightly packed) broccoli sprouts
2 cups cooked lima beans
Salt and pepper to taste
¼ cup soy milk or nonfat milk

In a saucepan, sauté garlic, celery, potatoes, pepper, thyme, and marjoram in oil for 2–3 minutes. Add water and simmer for 15 minutes. Add corn, broccoli sprouts, and cooked beans and simmer 5 minutes. Add salt and pepper and stir in milk. Mix well and serve.

Day 5

BREAKFAST
Breakfast Brown Rice and Raisins✓
Orange or apple juice
Decaf tea

LUNCH
Soy "hot dog" on whole-wheat bun
Sauerkraut
Pinto beans flavored with salsa
Seltzer

DINNER
Whole-grain pasta with marinara sauce
✗Cauliflower, broccoli and brussels sprouts steamed and
served with Herb Dressing✓ (see recipe in Day 4)
Poached Pears✓
Hot herbal tea

SNACK
Fruit Smoothie✓ (see Smoothie recipes at end of menus,
page 131)

Breakfast Brown Rice and Raisins (serves 4)

This is a good recipe in which to use extra cooked brown
rice.

3 cups cooked brown rice
½ cup raisins
¼ cup maple syrup
1 cup rice milk
½ cup chopped nuts
1 teaspoon ground cinnamon
½ teaspoon ground cardamom

Place all ingredients in a saucepan and bring to a boil over medium heat. Immediately reduce heat to low and allow mixture to simmer as you stir frequently for 5–8 minutes. Spoon into serving bowls and serve hot.

Poached Pears (serves 4)

 2½ cups apple juice
 Juice and zest of 1 lemon
 4 firm Bosc pears
 1 tablespoon fennel seeds

Mix apple juice and lemon in saucepan. Peel and core pears and add pears and peelings in the pan. Bring to a boil, then reduce heat and let pears cook for 3–5 minutes. Remove pears and chill. Strain liquid and return to pot with fennel and lemon zest. Cook on medium heat for 10 minutes or until thickened. Pears can be heated in sauce or served cold with warm sauce.

Day 6

BREAKFAST
 Fruity French Toast✓
 Orange juice
 Herbal tea

LUNCH
 Nutty Roast Loaf✓ (leftovers) in whole-wheat pita,
  topped with lettuce, tomato, and other favorite sand-
  wich veggies (recipe in Day 4)
 Seasonal fresh fruit
 Iced herbal tea

DINNER
 ✗Sprout It Out Salad✓
 Petite Red and Green Pasta✓
 Garlic bread
 Decaf tea

SNACK
  Hummus✓ and baked tortilla chips or raw vegetables

Fruity French Toast (serves 2)

  1 banana, peeled
  4 strawberries, or ⅓ cup blueberries or raspberries
  ⅓ cup apple juice
  4 slices whole-wheat or 7-grain bread
  ½ teaspoon cinnamon

Place the fruit, cinnamon, and juice in a blender and pulse until smooth. Soak the bread in the mixture and brown on both sides on a nonstick griddle or one sprayed with oil.

✗Sprout It Out Salad (serves 2–4)

  1 cup broccoli sprouts
  1 cup alfalfa sprouts
  1 cup mung bean sprouts
  2 cups shredded red cabbage
  Nutritional yeast

Mix sprouts and cabbage together in a bowl. Serve with Herb Dressing to taste (see recipe on page 104) and sprinkle with nutritional yeast.

Petite Red and Green Pasta (serves 4)

  10 ounces small pasta shells
  1 tablespoon olive oil
  2 cloves garlic, minced
  1 pound greens (kale, chard, dandelion, beet) with stems
    removed and leaves torn into 2-inch pieces (about 4
    cups)
  3 cups chopped fresh tomatoes
  1 tablespoon red wine vinegar
  1 teaspoon dried basil leaves (or 2 teaspoons fresh basil)

Prepare pasta according to package directions. Drain. In a nonstick skillet, heat oil with garlic and cook 1–2 minutes over medium heat. Add the greens, increase the heat, and cook, stirring constantly, until just wilted (4–5 minutes). Add the pasta, tomatoes, vinegar, and basil. Heat through and serve promptly.

Hummus (makes 2 cups)

2 cups cooked garbanzo beans
⅛ cup tahini
1 tablespoon olive oil
2 cloves garlic, minced
1 tablespoon lemon juice
½ teaspoon each cumin and coriander seed
Salt to taste

Combine all ingredients in food processor or blender and process until smooth. Use as a dip or sandwich spread.

Day 7

BREAKFAST
Buckwheat pancakes with fresh fruit
Apple juice
Herbal tea

LUNCH
✗Great Garbanzo Spread✓ on whole-grain pita or whole-wheat tortilla wrap with tomato, cucumber, and broccoli sprouts
Rockin' Moroccan Soup✓
Iced decaf tea

DINNER
Baked Salmon With Peppers and Mushrooms✓ or "Chick" Pasta with Broccoli and Mushrooms✓
✗Two Potato Scramble✓
Steamed fresh spinach
Cranapple Pudding✓
Hot tea

SNACK
   Nondairy frozen dessert

Great Garbanzo Spread *(makes 2 cups)*

   3 cups cooked garbanzo beans
   1 tablespoon lemon juice
   1/4 teaspoon each basil, garlic powder, ground cumin
   1 teaspoon onion powder
   1 tablespoon chopped coriander

Blend the beans in a blender or food processor. Add the remaining ingredients and mix well. Let stand for 1 hour at room temperature to allow the full flavor to come through.

Rockin' Moroccan Soup *(6–8 servings)*

   1 cup dried lima beans
   1 onion, chopped
   8 cups vegetable bouillon
   1 cup brown rice or cracked wheat
   1/2 cup raisins
   1 cup dried apricots, halved
   1 carrot, sliced
   2 stalks celery, cut into 1-inch chunks
   1/2 pound cabbage, chopped
   1/4 cup yellow split peas
   1 teaspoon cinnamon
   2 teaspoons sugar
   1 tablespoon lemon juice

Soak lima beans overnight; drain and rinse. Bring lima beans, onion, and bouillon to a boil and simmer 30 minutes. Add the brown rice or cracked wheat and cook 20 minutes. Add the remaining ingredients and simmer 25 minutes or until beans are tender.

Baked Salmon with Peppers and Mushrooms (serves 4)

1 cup red onion, sliced thin
4 peppers (mixture of green, red, and yellow), sliced in thin strips
4 cloves garlic, minced
1 cup shiitake mushrooms, sliced thin
4 salmon filets (5 ounces each)
½ cup dry white wine or ½ cup vegetable broth
2 tablespoons fresh lemon juice
½ teaspoon ground black pepper

Preheat oven to 450°. Combine the onion, peppers, garlic, and mushrooms in a baking dish. Place the salmon filets on top. Mix together the wine, lemon juice, and pepper and pour over the fish. Cover tightly with foil and make a few small holes in the foil. Bake for about 20 minutes, until fish is cooked through.

"Chick" Pasta with Broccoli and Mushrooms (serves 2)

½ tablespoon olive oil or other vegetable oil
1 teaspoon fennel seeds (optional)
¼ cup chopped almonds (optional)
1 cup diced tomatoes
1 red, yellow, or green pepper, roasted
½ cup chopped basil (or 1 teaspoon dried)
1 15-ounce can chickpeas (garbanzo beans), undrained
1 cup fresh broccoli, chopped into small pieces
½ cup sliced shiitake mushrooms
4 ounces of cooked pasta

Toast fennel seeds and almonds with the oil in a large skillet. Add the tomatoes, pepper, basil, chickpeas, broccoli, and mushrooms and cook over low heat until the broccoli is tender. Serve over cooked pasta.

✗Two Potato Scramble (serves 3–4)

1 medium yellow onion
2 carrots, sliced thin
½ cup water
2 white potatoes, sliced thin
1 sweet potato, sliced thin
½ pound fresh mushrooms, sliced
½ cup (lightly packed) broccoli sprouts, chopped
½ tablespoon low-salt soy sauce (optional)

Cook the onion and carrots in the water for 5 minutes. Add the potatoes and mix well. Cover the pan to steam for about 15 minutes, stirring occasionally. Add more water if needed. Add the mushrooms, broccoli sprouts, and soy sauce. Steam for 5 more minutes or until potatoes are tender.

Cranapple Pudding (serves 4–6)

2 tart apples, peeled, cored, and grated
4 cups whole-grain bread, cubed
2½ cups soy milk or nonfat milk
½ cup cranberries
½ cup raisins or currants
¼ cup plus 3 tablespoons pure maple syrup
1 tablespoon arrowroot
1½ teaspoons ground cinnamon
½ teaspoon salt
1 cup chopped walnuts

Preheat oven to 350°. In a large bowl, combine apples, bread, salt, milk, cranberries, raisins or currants, ¼ cup syrup, arrowroot, and 1 teaspoon cinnamon. Stir well and spoon mixture into a 2-quart baking dish. Place the remaining cinnamon, nuts, and 3 tablespoons of syrup in a food processor and pulse until coarsely chopped. Sprinkle this mixture over the pudding. Bake for 45 minutes. Let cool for at least 20 minutes before serving.

Day 8

BREAKFAST
Fruit Smoothie✓ (see Smoothie recipes at end of menus, page 131)
Rainbow Cornbread✓
Herbal tea

LUNCH
Chickpea Gumbo✓
Whole-grain roll
Flavored seltzer

DINNER
✗Sprout-About✓ served over brown rice or whole-wheat toast
✗Raw spinach salad with radishes, cucumber, onion, mushrooms, broccoli sprouts, avocado, and Herb Dressing✓ (see Day 5)
Wheatberry Delight✓
Herbal tea

SNACK
Peanut butter or almond butter on rye crackers

Rainbow Cornbread *(serves 8)*

1 cup cornmeal
1 cup whole-wheat flour
1 tablespoon baking powder
1 tablespoon honey
1½ cups warm water
Any combination of the following to equal ½ cup: finely chopped onion; green, yellow, and red pepper; pimientos; grated carrot or zucchini

Preheat oven to 375°. Mix dry ingredients in a bowl. In another bowl, mix honey and warm water, then add to dry ingredients and fold in vegetables. Stir until mixed. Pour into nonstick 8-inch baking dish. Bake for 20 minutes.

Chickpea Gumbo (serves 6–8)

- 1 onion, chopped
- 2 cloves garlic, minced
- 1 green pepper, chopped
- 1 28-ounce can plum tomatoes, chopped (save juice)
- 1 dried red pepper, crumbled
- ¼ cup flour plus ¼ cup cold water (optional, to thicken the gumbo)
- 1 pound okra, sliced
- ¼ cup parsley, chopped
- ¼ cup fresh basil leaves, chopped
- 1 bay leaf
- 2 cans chickpeas, undrained
- 1 tablespoon lemon juice

Bring onion, garlic, pepper, tomatoes and their liquid, and red pepper to a boil in a large pot and simmer 20 minutes. If you like thick gumbo, stir flour into the water and whisk it into the hot stew. Stir in the remaining ingredients and simmer 10 minutes. Serve the gumbo over brown rice if desired.

✗Sprout-About (serves 4)

- 1 pound firm tofu, frozen and thawed, then crumbled (or 12 ounces shredded chicken breast)
- 1 small leek, chopped
- 1 clove garlic, minced
- 1 tablespoon olive oil
- 2 tablespoons soy sauce
- 2 tomatoes, chopped
- 2 cups (lightly packed) broccoli sprouts
- 2 teaspoons arrowroot
- Salt and pepper to taste

In a skillet, sauté the tofu (or chicken), leek, and garlic in oil and soy sauce for 3–4 minutes. Add the tomatoes and sprouts and sauté the mixture for 5 minutes. Dissolve the arrowroot in a small amount of water and pour over the mixture in the skillet, stirring constantly. Season with salt and pepper to taste. Serve over brown rice or whole-wheat toast.

Wheatberry Delight (serves 4–6)

1½ cups wheatberries
¼ cup soy or rice milk (or nonfat milk)
3 tablespoons pure maple syrup
4 dried apricots, chopped
¼ cup dried currants or raisins
Dash of salt
¼ cup crushed almonds (optional)

Place wheatberries in a saucepan, cover with water, and simmer until tender, about 30 minutes. Drain. Add milk and bring to a boil. Reduce heat to low and simmer 5 minutes. Add remaining ingredients except nuts and simmer for 2–3 minutes. Remove from heat and top with almonds, if desired. Serve hot.

Day 9

BREAKFAST
Oatmeal with raisins and/or chopped nuts and sprinkled with wheat germ
½ bagel with all-fruit jelly
Grapefruit juice
Hot decaf tea

LUNCH
✗Crazy Curried Carrot Soup✓
Whole-grain crackers
Vegetable juice

DINNER
Billion Bean Chili✓
Rainbow Cornbread✓ (leftover; see Day 8)

Steamed carrots
Flavored seltzer

SNACK
Handful each dry-roasted nuts and raisins

✗Crazy Curried Carrot Soup (serves 6)

5 cups carrots, peeled and cut into 1-inch pieces
1 cup turnips, peeled and cut into 1-inch pieces
5 cups vegetable broth
4 teaspoons minced fresh ginger
1 teaspoon each curry powder and ground cumin
½ teaspoon ground black pepper
3 cloves garlic, minced
1 cup (lightly packed) broccoli sprouts, finely chopped
3 tablespoons chopped fresh cilantro leaves

Combine all ingredients except the cilantro and broccoli sprouts in a saucepan and bring to a boil. Reduce heat to low and simmer for 30 minutes. Place the mixture in a blender or food processor, 2 to 3 cups at a time, add chopped sprouts, and blend until smooth. Return the blended mixture to the pan and reheat. Stir in cilantro and serve.

Billion Bean Chili (serves 4–6)

Mix up your favorite beans in this hearty chili. Make a double batch and freeze some in small containers for a quick lunch or dinner.

1 cup each chopped onion, diced carrot, diced celery
1 cup water
3 cloves garlic, minced
½ cup chopped green, red, or yellow pepper
1½ tablespoons chili powder
1 14-ounce block of extra-firm tofu or 2 veggie burgers, crumbled
½ teaspoon cayenne

2 teaspoons mustard
2 28-ounce cans crushed tomatoes (save the juice)
5 cups of cooked beans, any combination of kidney,
    pinto, soy, black, navy, adzuki
Salt to taste

In a large saucepan, simmer onion in 1 cup water over medium heat until the onion is translucent. Add the garlic, carrot, celery, pepper, chili powder, tofu or veggie burger, and cayenne. Simmer and stir for 2 minutes. Add the tomatoes and stir until the sauce is well blended and then add the beans. Lower heat and simmer for 40 minutes. Add the mustard and salt and simmer for 5 minutes.

Day 10

BREAKFAST
Scrambled Morning✓
Tempting Tempeh Strips✓
Apple juice
Coffee substitute

LUNCH
✗Where's the Chicken Soup✓
Whole-grain crackers
Iced decaf tea

DINNER
✗Stuffed Sprouted Shells✓ with Sprout Pasta Sauce✓
Steamed zucchini
Whole-grain roll with soy margarine
Hot decaf tea

SNACK
Air-popped popcorn with nutritional yeast

Scrambled Morning *(serves 4)*

2 tablespoons olive oil (optional; you can steam the vegetables)
1 pound extra-firm tofu, cubed
1 medium onion, chopped
1 medium zucchini, cut into ½-inch-thick circles
4 ounces asparagus, cut into 1-inch pieces
2 garlic cloves, minced
2 medium tomatoes, cut into ½-inch cubes
2 tablespoons tamari
1 teaspoon ground cumin

In a large frying pan, heat oil over medium-high heat. Or add ⅛ cup water and steam the tofu, onion, zucchini, asparagus, and garlic. Stir-fry until crisp, about 3 minutes. Add tomatoes, tamari, and cumin and heat through, about 1 minute. Serve immediately.

Tempting Tempeh Strips *(makes 12-16 strips)*

Spray oil
8 ounces tempeh, sliced into thin strips
¼ cup brown rice syrup
2 tablespoons soy sauce
1 tablespoon mustard
Pepper to taste

Preheat oven to 450°. Lightly spray oil on a baking sheet and place strips of tempeh on sheet. Drizzle with syrup and soy sauce and dot with mustard. Season with pepper and lightly spray the sheet again. Bake for 5–10 minutes, until lightly browned. Turn strips over and bake for another 5 minutes.

✗Where's the Chicken Soup *(serves 6)*

½ pound firm tofu, frozen and then thawed; or 8 ounces cooked chicken, diced
2 cups noodles

    5 cups vegetable broth
    1 carrot, chopped
    1 stalk celery, chopped
    1 onion, chopped
    ½ cup (lightly packed) broccoli sprouts
    2 cloves garlic, minced
    ½ teaspoon each dried marjoram, dried thyme, sage
    1 cup peas, fresh or frozen and thawed
    ½ cup chopped fresh parsley

*Gently squeeze the water from the thawed tofu and cut into
½-inch cubes. In a large pot, cook the noodles in water until
tender. Drain and set aside in a bowl. In the same pot, combine the broth, carrot, celery, onion, sprouts, garlic, and seasonings. Simmer over medium heat for 5 minutes. Stir in the
tofu, peas, and parsley and simmer for another 2 minutes. Add
the noodles, allow to reach a simmer, and remove from heat.*

✗Stuffed Sprouted Shells (serves 4)

    8 ounces large pasta shells, cooked according to package
        directions
    2½ cups broccoli sprouts
    ½ cup mashed tofu (or nonfat cottage cheese)
    1 tablespoon nutritional yeast
    2 tablespoons soy sauce

*Preheat oven to 425°. While pasta is cooking, place other
ingredients in a bowl and mix together thoroughly. Drain the
pasta and stuff the shells with the mixture. Place the shells in
a nonstick baking dish and top with your favorite tomato sauce
or use the Sprout Pasta Sauce recipe. Bake for 20 minutes.*

✗Sprout Pasta Sauce

    1 cup water
    1 onion, minced
    1½ cups crushed tomatoes
    2 cloves garlic, minced

1 cup broccoli sprouts
2 teaspoons arrowroot
3 tablespoons tomato purée
1 tablespoon soy sauce
¼ teaspoon thyme
Salt to taste

In a saucepan mix together ¾ cup water with the onion, tomatoes, garlic, and sprouts. Boil for 3–5 minutes. Dissolve the arrowroot in ¼ cup water mixed with the tomato purée and the soy sauce. Season with thyme and salt to taste. Combine all ingredients and serve over pasta.

Day 11

BREAKFAST
Fruit Smoothie✓ (see Smoothie recipes at end of menus, page 131)
English muffin with all-fruit jelly or peanut butter
Hot decaf tea

LUNCH
✗Potato Lentil Burger✓ on whole-grain roll with sprouts, onion, and tomato
Baked tortilla chips with salsa
Flavored seltzer

DINNER
Barbecued Tofu✓ (or 3 ounces barbecued chicken breast)
Corny Couscous Salad✓
✗Swiss Chard, Chickpeas, and Sprouts✓
Coffee substitute

SNACK
Nondairy frozen dessert

✗Potato Lentil Burgers (makes 4 burgers)

¼ cup chopped onion
¼ cup chopped celery
¼ cup water
1 cup cooked lentils
1 cup mashed potatoes
½ cup bread crumbs
½ teaspoon each dried marjoram, sage, parsley, thyme
Broccoli sprouts
Tomato slices
Onion slices

Preheat oven to 350°. Sauté onion and celery in water for 10 minutes. Combine remaining ingredients except sprouts and tomato and onion slices in a bowl and mix well. Form into patties and place on nonstick baking sheet. Bake for 15–20 minutes each side. Serve on whole-wheat roll or pita with broccoli sprouts and tomato and onion slices.

Barbecued Tofu (serves 4)

1 pound extra-firm tofu, well drained
1 teaspoon each salt and pepper
1 tablespoon honey
¼ teaspoon cayenne
1 teaspoon chili powder
2 cloves garlic, mashed
2 tablespoons organic ketchup
½ cup apple cider vinegar

Preheat oven to 300°. Cut the tofu into ½-inch cubes. Combine the remaining ingredients in a large bowl, mix well, and add the tofu. Use a rubber spatula to gently mix the tofu in the marinade. Place tofu and marinade in a baking dish and bake uncovered for 45 minutes, tossing tofu one or two times during baking. Serve hot.

Corny Couscous Salad (serves 2-4)

1 cup water
⅔ cup uncooked couscous
1 cup corn kernels
1 cup chopped tomatoes
½ cup chopped green pepper
¼ cup minced onion
⅛ cup finely chopped fresh cilantro or parsley

Dressing:
2 tablespoons each wine vinegar, water, and low-sodium soy sauce
½ teaspoon Dijon mustard
Tabasco sauce to taste (optional)

Boil the water, turn off the heat, and add the couscous. Let sit for 5–10 minutes until the water is absorbed. Place the corn, tomatoes, pepper, onion, and cilantro or parsley in a serving bowl with the couscous. In a small jar or bowl, mix the dressing ingredients and blend. Pour dressing over the salad and mix well. For best flavor, cover and chill for at least 2 hours.

✗Swiss Chard, Chickpeas, and Sprouts (serves 6–8)

2 pounds Swiss chard, chopped and washed
6 cloves garlic, mashed
2 tablespoons salsa
2 teaspoons ground coriander
Salt and pepper to taste
1 cup minced onion
2 15-ounce cans chickpeas (save liquid)
1 cup (lightly packed) broccoli sprouts
Lemon wedges (optional)

In a large pot, steam Swiss chard in a small amount of water, if needed, until tender, about 5 minutes. Drain and set aside.

In a small bowl, mix together garlic, salsa, coriander, and salt and pepper. Set aside. In a large skillet, sauté onion in a small amount of water for 6–7 minutes. Add garlic mixture and mix well. Add chard, chickpeas (with liquid), and sprouts. Stir and cook until heated through, about 10 minutes. Serve with lemon wedges, if desired.

Day 12

BREAKFAST

 Three-Grain Cereal✓
 Mixed fresh fruit with yogurt (optional)
 Decaf tea

LUNCH

 How Green Is My Garden Soup✓
 ✗Avocado, tomato, cucumber, and sprout sandwich on
  whole-wheat tortilla or pita
 Iced tea

DINNER

 Split Pea and Vegetable Stew✓
 ✗Sassy Sprout Salad✓
 Whole-wheat bread
 Flavored seltzer

SNACK

 Fruit Smoothie✓ (see Smoothie recipes at end of menus,
  page 131)

Three-Grain Cereal (serves 4)

 2 cups no-fat soy milk (or nonfat milk)
 1 cup water
 ½ teaspoon salt
 ¼ cup cream of buckwheat
 ¼ cup wheat flakes
 2 tablespoons millet
 Honey or maple syrup (optional)

In a medium saucepan, combine milk, water, and salt. Stir in remaining ingredients. Bring to a boil, stirring frequently. Reduce heat to low and simmer for 12–15 minutes, stirring occasionally. Spoon into bowls and top with honey or maple syrup, if desired.

How Green Is My Garden Soup (4–6 servings)

    2 onions, chopped
    4 cloves garlic, minced
    1 green pepper, chopped
    4 cups vegetable bouillon
    ½ cup bulgur
    1 28-ounce can plum tomatoes, chopped
    1 dried red pepper, crumbled
    1 head romaine lettuce, shredded
    1 cup each chopped parsley, chopped fresh basil leaves,
        baby lima beans, diced zucchini, and peas

Bring onions, garlic, green pepper, and ½ cup bouillon to a boil. Simmer about 10 minutes. Add the remaining bouillon, bulgur, tomatoes and red pepper and simmer 30 minutes. Add the lettuce, parsley, basil, lima beans, zucchini, and peas and cook 10 minutes.

Split Pea and Vegetable Stew (serves 4)

    1 cup dry green split peas
    3 cups water
    ¼ pound each green beans cut into 1-inch lengths,
        chopped zucchini, and sliced mushrooms,
    1 green pepper, chopped
    1 tablespoon soy sauce
    1 teaspoon mustard

Combine split peas and water. Bring to a boil, reduce heat, cover, and simmer 1 hour. Steam all other vegetables separately until tender. Combine the cooked split peas and vegetables. Stir in soy sauce and mustard.

✗Sassy Sprout Salad (serves 4)

1 cup each alfalfa sprouts, broccoli sprouts, and mung
bean sprouts
2 green onions, chopped
1 carrot, shredded
1 red pepper, chopped
¼ cup chopped pimiento
1 tablespoon cider vinegar
1 tablespoon tamari
2 teaspoons lemon juice

*Combine sprouts and vegetables in a large bowl. Combine
the vinegar, tamari, and lemon juice in a cup and stir. Pour
over the sprouts and vegetables, cover, and chill for one hour.*

Day 13

BREAKFAST
Up With the Sun Quinoa✓
Honeydew or cantaloupe
English muffin with all-fruit jelly
Herbal tea

LUNCH
Millet Croquettes or Loaf✓ on whole-wheat toast
Steamed mustard greens with lemon
Iced tea

DINNER
✗Hurry Scurry Hot Pot Curry✓ served over quinoa, rice,
or whole-wheat toast
✗Raw spinach salad with cucumbers, sprouts, and toma-
toes with lemon
Vegetable juice

SNACK
✗White Bean Spread✓ with raw vegetables

Up with the Sun Quinoa *(serves 4)*

3 cups cooked quinoa
3 apricots, coarsely chopped
1 orange, peeled and sectioned
1 cup seedless red grapes, halved
¼ cup raisins
Cinnamon, if desired

Combine all ingredients in a bowl and chill for 1 hour or overnight.

Millet Croquettes or Loaf *(serves 4)*

1½ cups millet, well rinsed
3 large carrots, sliced or 1 medium butternut squash, peeled and sliced
1 onion, sliced
4½ cups water

Combine all ingredients in a large quart saucepan. Boil and then simmer covered for 20 minutes. For a loaf, transfer the hot mix into a loaf pan. When cool, slice and serve with hot gravy or a favorite sauce. For croquettes: When the mixture is cool enough to handle, shape into patties or balls and fry.

✗Hurry Scurry Hot Pot Curry *(serves 4)*

2 tablespoons olive oil
3–6 teaspoons (to taste) curry powder
2 cups (lightly packed) broccoli sprouts
4 sweet potatoes, peeled and shredded
1½ cups cauliflower florets
1 cup peas
1¼ cups plain soy yogurt (or nonfat yogurt)
1 banana, sliced
Crushed cashew nuts, if desired

In a large saucepan, heat oil, 3 teaspoons curry powder, sprouts, potatoes, and cauliflower. Add enough water to allow the mixture to simmer for 15–20 minutes. Add the peas, remove the pan from the heat, and stir in the yogurt. Add the banana and mix in the nuts if desired. Return to heat, add the remaining curry (to taste), and heat. Allow to stand for a few minutes before serving. Serve over rice, couscous, quinoa, or whole wheat toast.

✗White Bean Spread (makes 2–3 sandwiches or about 1 cup)

 1 small onion, chopped
 2 small cloves garlic, minced
 1½ cups cooked white beans or kidney beans
 2 teaspoons soy sauce
 2 tablespoons apple juice
 ½ teaspoon chili powder
 Broccoli sprouts, tomato slices, and cucumber slices for
   garnish

Place the onion and garlic in a saucepan with a small amount of water and cook until the onion is soft. Add the beans and mash them as they heat. Add chili powder, soy sauce and apple juice. Stir well. Put in a bowl and refrigerate for several hours. Use as a sandwich spread and top with broccoli sprouts and tomato and cucumber slices. Also can be used as a dip for raw vegetables.

Day 14

BREAKFAST
  Berry Merry Breakfast✓
  English muffin with all-fruit jelly
  Orange or grapefruit juice
  Herbal tea

LUNCH
  ✗Black-Eyed Sprout Soup✓
  Rice cakes with all-fruit jelly
  Coffee substitute

DINNER
  Stuffed Peppers✓
  Purple-Top Puree✓
  ✗Green salad with tomatoes, peppers, onion, mushrooms,
    sprouts, radishes, and other fresh vegetables of your
    choice
  Herbal tea

SNACK
  Millet Apple Raisin Bar✓

Berry Merry Breakfast (serves 2)

  1 pint fresh strawberries
  1 mango, peeled and cut into pieces
  5 ice cubes
  1 tablespoon chopped fresh mint leaves
  1 cup soy yogurt (or nonfat plain yogurt)
  1 teaspoon pure maple syrup (optional)

*Combine all ingredients in a blender or food processor and
blend until ice is crushed.*

✗Black-Eyed Sprout Soup (serves 3)

This is a good way to use leftover cooked rice and black-
eyed peas.

  1 cup water
  2 cups vegetable broth
  1 cup onion, chopped
  ½ cup cooked black-eyed peas
  ½ cup broccoli sprouts
  ½ cup lentil sprouts
  ¼ cup cooked brown rice

In a saucepan, simmer the onion in the water and broth for 3–4 minutes. Add the peas and bring to a boil. Remove from the heat and add the rice and sprouts just before serving.

Stuffed Peppers (serves 4)

- 1 onion, diced
- ½ cup celery, chopped
- ¼ pound mushrooms, chopped
- ¼ cup water
- 1 cup nonfat tomato sauce
- 1 cup cooked brown rice
- ½ cup corn
- 1 teaspoon sage
- ¼ teaspoon dried basil or ½ teaspoon fresh basil
- ¼ teaspoon garlic powder
- 4 large green peppers, cored

Preheat oven to 375°. In a small skillet, cook onion, celery, and mushrooms in water for about 15 minutes. Stir in ½ cup tomato sauce, rice, corn, and seasonings. Stuff the rice mixture into the peppers, and place the peppers in a baking dish. Pour the remaining tomato sauce over the peppers and add 1 cup of water to the baking dish to prevent the peppers from drying out. Cover and bake for 45 minutes. Uncover and bake an additional 10–15 minutes.

Purple-Top Puree (serves 4)

- 3 purple-top turnips (1½ pounds) peeled and cut into 1-inch pieces
- 2 large potatoes (1½ pounds) peeled and cut into 1-inch pieces
- 2 medium carrots, cut into ½-inch slices
- ¼ cup (packed) fresh parsley, chopped
- ½ teaspoon ground black pepper
- Salt to taste

Steam turnips, potatoes, and carrots in a steamer basket until tender, about 10–15 minutes. Drain well. Place turnips, pota-

toes, parsley, pepper, and salt in a food processor. Purée until smooth. Stir in carrot slices. Reheat if needed.

Millet Apple Raisin Bars

    1 cup millet, rinsed well and drained
    3 cups apple juice (or your favorite juice)
    1 cup raisins
    Pinch of salt
    1 teaspoon vanilla (optional)

Combine all ingredients (except vanilla) in a stock pot, bring to a boil, then lower heat and simmer about 20 minutes. Remove from heat, stir well, add vanilla, and pour the mixture into a cake pan. Let it cool, then slice and serve like brownies.

Fruit Smoothies

Each recipe is for one serving.

- Mango Morning: 1 banana, 1 mango (peeled and pitted), and 8 ounces orange juice
- Strawberry Surprise: 5–6 large strawberries (tops removed), 1 banana, 8 ounces apple juice
- Awesome Apple: ¼ cup applesauce, 1 teaspoon cinnamon, 1 banana, 8 ounces apple juice
- Great Guava Grapefruit: 1 guava (peeled and pitted), ½ banana, 8 ounces grapefruit juice

Place all ingredients in a blender or food processor and blend until smooth. If you don't have these appliances, mash the fruits well and place them in a jar with a tight lid. Shake vigorously.

8. Other Ways to Reduce Your Risk of Cancer

WHEN YOU FOLLOW A HEALTHFUL, CANCER-PREVENTION EATing plan, you give your body a good environment in which to function. Nutritious food is just one component of a cancer- and disease-preventive lifestyle, and broccoli sprouts can be an important part of that effort. Just as your body, mind, and spirit all coexist and work together to make you who you are, so do a variety of internal and external factors exist that can have either a beneficial or detrimental effect on your overall health. When we look at ways to reduce the risk of cancer, the areas to consider include: alcohol use, smoking, obesity, exercise, environmental toxins and conditions, and genetics. In this chapter you'll learn about the latest research on the commonly known cancer risks and how you can avoid them and/or prevent their influence on your health. This chapter is not meant to scare you but to give you some tools to better protect you and your family.

ALCOHOL USE

A link between alcohol and cancer has been known since the late 1950s, when researchers reported on the special relationship between alcohol and colorectal cancer. Since then, many studies have supported the claim that moderate alcohol consumption can increase the risk of cancer. What is meant by "moderate"? According to the American Cancer Institute Human Nutrition Information Service at the United States Department of Agriculture, and the American Institute for Cancer Research, it means one serving of alcohol (1 ounce of hard liquor, 12 ounces of beer, or 6 ounces of wine) per day for women and two servings for men. In one study, Dr. Matthew Longnecker of the University of California at Los Angeles evaluated thirty-eight studies of alcohol and breast cancer. He determined that the risk of breast cancer increased 10 percent among women who had one drink a day and 25 percent among those who had two drinks per day. Alcohol increases the amount of estradiol the body manufactures, and this in turn stimulates breast cancer growth.

Yet some studies indicate that moderate alcohol use may actually be beneficial for women who are older than fifty and who have various risk factors for heart disease. So do the benefits outweigh the downfalls? Not likely. According to the International Agency for Research on Cancer in 1988, "There is sufficient evidence to suggest that alcoholic beverages are carcinogens to humans." In this capacity, alcohol use can contribute significantly to the development of mouth, larynx, pharynx, esophagus, liver, colorectal, and breast cancers. Here are a few ways alcohol contributes to cancer:

- Alcohol causes cell damage, which promotes cell division. The stimulation of cell division can be a factor in the development of cancer.

- Some carcinogens are activated by enzymes, and alcohol stimulates some of these enzymes.

- The body's ability to fight damage from free radicals is reduced by alcohol consumption.

- Some alcoholic beverages contain carcinogens. For example, beer contains nitrosamines; bourbon, sherry, fruity brandies, and other beverages contain urethane.

- Irritation of the lining of the mouth, esophagus, and

throat by alcohol or other substances has been linked to
of these organs.

If you drink alcohol and smoke, your risk for cancer
increases dramatically. Your chances of developing liver
cancer are fourteen times greater if you smoke and drink
heavily. One study even suggests that moderate drinking
along with smoking increases the chances of getting neck
and head cancers fifteenfold.

The best cancer-prevention approach with alcohol is to
avoid it. Barring that, limit your drinks to no more than three
or four a week. If you are often in situations where drinking is
acceptable and encouraged, order mineral water, flavored
seltzer alone or with fruit juice, or a nonalcoholic beer or wine.
To reduce stomach irritation from alcohol, eat both before you
drink and while you drink. And when you are thirsty, especially on a hot day, resist the temptation to guzzle down a beer.
Instead, reach for a glass of water, seltzer, or juice.

Alcohol abuse, which is defined as drinking more than two
alcoholic beverages per day, can be treated successfully. Help
can come in the form of support groups such as Alcoholics
Anonymous and similar peer-counseling organizations, individual counseling, or treatment facilities for substance abuse.
For information about these approaches, contact the nearest
AA group listed in your telephone directory; or call the Center
for Substance Abuse Treatment Referral at 1-800-662-HELP.

SMOKING

Despite the fact that smoking kills more than 435,000 Americans every year, 46 million Americans still light up every
day. Even though each cigarette they smoke reduces their
life by seven minutes and they know smoking causes cancer,
they keep reaching for another and another.

The addictive power of tobacco is hard, but not impossible, to shake. The arguments against smoking are certainly
food for thought.

- Smoking is associated not only with lung cancer but also with laryngeal, oral, esophageal, urinary, bladder, kidney, pancreatic, and cervical cancers.

- Tobacco use increases your chances of dying not only from cancer but also from chronic bronchitis, heart disease, emphysema, and heart attack.

- Smoking promotes premature wrinkling, peptic ulcers, and dental and gum disease.

- Children with parents who smoke are twice as likely to become smokers themselves.

- Pregnant women who smoke have increased chances of experiencing a miscarriage, stillbirth, premature birth, or low-birth-weight baby.

- Secondhand smoke has higher concentrations of carcinogens than does mainstream smoke.

- Smoking costs Americans $65 billion a year in health-care-related costs and lost productivity.

Tobacco "Bad Guys"

More than four thousand chemical compounds are in tobacco smoke, and forty-three of them are known carcinogens. Nicotine leads the pack of tars and gases, such as carbon monoxide, to do dirty work in the lungs and throughout the body. From the moment you inhale, it takes only seven seconds for the toxic substances in tobacco smoke to go through the lungs into the bloodstream and to the brain. The brain signals the nerve endings to respond to the stress of these foreign substances by releasing substances called catecholamines. The catecholamines in turn reduce the flow of oxygen and blood throughout the body. The lack of adequate oxygen causes the heart to pump harder and faster and leaves the blood deprived of oxygen.

In the lungs, the inhaled tars stick to the lung lining and eventually kill the cilia, the tiny hairs that help keep the lungs clear. When the cilia are gone, the lungs become a gathering place for the tumor-causing substances inhaled with the tobacco smoke. Only about 10 percent of inhaled toxins leave the body; the remainder stay in the lungs to do their damage.

How to Quit

If you smoke and want to quit, you can join the three million Americans each year who kick the tobacco habit. How you choose to quit is up to you; what works for your spouse or coworker may not work for you. Here are the most common stop-smoking techniques:

Cold Turkey.

Many experts say that this is the most effective way to leave the nicotine habit behind you forever. It can cause more severe side effects than other methods, but if they are anticipated and planned for, their severity can be greatly lessened. For example:

- Anxiety and irritability. Plan relaxing, "just for you" activities, such as meditation, long hot baths, deep breathing exercises, or walks with friends.

- Dry mouth. Your body will produce less mucus, which may leave your mouth dry. Keep a bottle of water handy, or keep chewing gum or sugar-free hard candy with you.

- Coughing. About 20 percent of people who stop smoking cough more than they did when they smoked. This is a temporary condition and is actually a cleansing process. As the cilia in the lungs recover, the body attempts to eliminate phlegm. Drinking warm tea or sucking on sugar-free cough drops can help.

- Constipation. Drink eight glasses of water a day and follow the dietary plan outlined in Chapter 4. Eating the recommended amount of fruits, vegetables, and grains is especially important to keep your bowel movements regular.

Gradual Withdrawal.

If going cold turkey sounds like more than you can handle, a gradual tapering off of cigarettes or postponing your next smoke may be a better method for you. Choose a withdrawal strategy and stick with it. If you smoke two packs a day now, you may decide to reduce the number of cigarettes you smoke a day by five. If you normally light up a cigarette the minute you get up in the morning, you could delay that cigarette for perhaps an hour. Every time you want a cigarette, delay it for an hour. When you've reduced the number of cigarettes to less than half of what you used to smoke, reduce that to half, and then quit altogether.

Nicotine-Replacement Products.

Nicotine gum and nicotine patches release nicotine into the body and taper the amount over time. These products are available by prescription and should be used under a doctor's guidance. Many people find the patch easier to use than the gum. There are several types of patches on the market, and you and your physician can choose the best plan for you. WARNING: When using a nicotine patch, do not smoke. You can suffer from an overdose of nicotine, which can trigger a fatal heart attack in some people.

Support Groups.

Walking away from any addiction can be extremely difficult for people who do not have the encouragement and support of their family, friends, and peers. Smoking-cessation groups, sponsored by health groups, employers, hospitals, or private businesses, provide these incentives for many people, including those who do have support from people close to them. Programs such as Fresh Start, Freedom From Smoking (sponsored by the American Lung Association), and Smokenders have sessions run by individuals trained to offer and help implement smoking cessation strategies. One major portion of these programs is behavior modification: making people aware of the automatic responses and habits they have built around smoking and then helping them change those behaviors. Some people, for example, always smoke while talking on the telephone, or when they drink a cup of coffee. Being aware of the triggers for smoking allows you to make both physical and mental adjustments to break that habit.

Hypnosis and Acupuncture.

One in four people who use hypnosis to quit smoking is smoke-free six months later. This quit rate is comparable to those obtained by other smoking-cessation methods. According to the American Society of Clinical Hypnosis, smokers need more than one session to effectively quit smoking and should stay away from anyone who claims that he or she can get you to quit after just one. This is a popular tactic taken by some hypnotherapists who do nationwide tours and hold one several-hour smoking cessation session in a city before moving on to another location. To find a reputable, licensed hypnotherapist, see Appendix A.

Acupuncture for smoking cessation involves inserting a tiny needle or staplelike object into the outer ear. Several sessions are usually necessary for success. For a list of certified acupuncturists, see Appendix A.

While You're Quitting: How to Cope

Quitting smoking may bring a few challenges your way, but they can be handled if you anticipate them. Here are a few problem areas and how to cope with them:

• **Weight Gain.** "Smoking keeps my weight down." "I'll get fat if I quit." Gaining weight is one of the biggest fears of people who quit smoking. Most ex-smokers, however, gain only five to ten pounds. Yet as soon as they put on a few extra pounds, some would-be ex-smokers decide to go on a diet, and the combined stress from trying to stop smoking and not eating usually causes them to fail at both. The best way to avoid gaining weight while also avoiding the temptation to smoke is to plan ahead. Avoid sugar and high-calorie foods by drinking flavored seltzer water or snacking on air-popped popcorn and crunchy vegetables. Stay away from acidic foods and liquids, such as citrus fruits and juices, tomatoes, vinegar, coffee, and nonherbal tea, because acidy foods increase your craving for nicotine. (Note: This is a temporary measure; you can return to eating these foods as the period of intense cravings subsides.) Carry bottled water with you and drink eight glasses of water a day. Water helps flush tobacco toxins from the body.

• **Stress.** For many people, the stress associated with quitting smoking is hard to handle. Suddenly other situations in their lives become unmanageable. Even waiting in line at the grocery store or having a flat tire can seem like a major catastrophe and send them reaching for a cigarette. If you know you tend to be impatient in certain situations, avoid them as much as possible during your withdrawal period. Take a different route home from work or go to the supermarket when it's less crowded. Consider learning some stress management techniques, such as yoga, meditation, deep-breathing exercises, and progressive relaxation. In fact, stress may be a contributing factor in cancer and has definitely been identified as contributing to heart disease, hypertension, and other medical conditions. Thus a stress management plan can protect you on more than one front!

• **Temptation and Habit.** During the initial withdrawal period, which can last weeks or months depending on the individual, you may need to avoid or alter situations that you associated with smoking. If you and your coworkers spend coffee breaks outside in a smoking area, take a refreshing walk instead. Some people even find it difficult at first to do routine tasks without a cigarette in their hand. Driving, talking on the phone, or watching television may be awkward or stressful at first. Bring water and hard sugarless candy with you in the car or sing with the radio. If you have a cassette or CD player in the car, play relaxing music or listen to books on tape. At home, set up a jigsaw puzzle next to the telephone or television to keep your hands occupied while talking on the phone or watching your favorite show. Take up a new hobby to keep your hands and mind occupied. Avoid settings that can tempt you into smoking, such as smoky bars or gatherings where people are smoking, or make it a point to stay with the nonsmokers. If you always have a cigarette after eating, brush your teeth instead. If having a cup of coffee triggers an intense craving for a cigarette, switch to tea or another beverage.

"Gotta Have a Cigarette." Many people who quit smoking, but not all, experience moderate to intense cravings for nicotine for weeks and even up to six months after quitting. When that happens, the American Cancer Society recommends the "four Ds": DELAY, DEEP breathing, DRINK a glass of water, and DO something, such as walking or yoga, or calling a friend for support.

Finally, let other people around you know that you have quit smoking. This helps you in two ways. One, they will know why you are irritable. And two, knowing that other people are counting on you to really stop smoking—or wanting to show them you really can do it—is good incentive to keep going.

HERE COMES THE SUN

Skin cancer is both the most prevalent form of cancer and the easiest to avoid. More than 730,000 Americans had skin cancer in 1994, and the incidence continues to rise. Between

1950 and 1985, malignant melanoma, the deadliest form of skin cancer, rose 500 percent. Much of the increase in skin cancer is attributed to people's fascination with the sun and suntans. Because of this sun worship, it is estimated that nearly 50 percent of men and women who reach age sixty-five will have skin cancer.

Types of Skin Cancer

The most common form of skin cancer is basal-cell carcinoma, which first appears as tiny, round, pearly lumps on the face, hands, or neck. These tumors usually grow very slowly and may take years to reach one-half inch in diameter. Left untreated, they can become crusty and bleed or form ulcers, or root under the skin and cause disfigurement. Basal-cell carcinoma rarely spreads to other parts of the body. When caught early, the cure rate is nearly 100 percent.

Squamous-cell carcinoma is the second most commonly seen skin cancer. It affects 130,000 people a year and is usually found on skin areas exposed to the sun: face, mouth, neck, hands, arms, back, ears, and lips. It appears as a raised red or pink scaly bump, or as a wartlike growth. Unlike basal-cell growths, squamous-cell carcinoma can spread rapidly and can affect other organs. It can be deadly, although early detection and treatment results in a 95 percent cure rate.

Malignant melanoma is less common but can be lethal. Some melanomas appear as new skin growths, or moles, but others take hold in an existing mole. Moles you are born with, called congenital moles, have a greater risk of becoming malignant than do new ones. Any change in a mole, such as appearance of irregular borders or a change in size or color should be examined immediately by a physician.

Risks for Skin Cancer and How to Prevent It

Certain skin types are at higher risk of developing skin cancer than others. People with any of the following factors or characteristics fall into this category:

- A fair complexion, blond or red hair, lots of freckles, and/or blue, green, or gray eyes

- A large (more than twenty-five) number of moles

- A family history of xeroderma pigmentosum, albinism, basal-cell nevus syndrome, melanoma, or dysplastic nevus syndrome

- Pregnancy, which increases a woman's sensitivity to sunlight

- Exposure to medical X rays or any treatments that include artificial UV radiation

- Exposure to chemicals such as arsenic and polycyclic aromatic hydrocarbons such as those found in asphalt, coal tars, pitch, paraffin waxes, and lubricating oils

- Use of psoralen (a drug to treat psoriasis), tetracycline, sulfa drugs, thiazide diuretic or indomethacin, or any medication that contains Retin-A increases sensitivity to ultraviolet light while these substances are being used

If any of these risks apply to you, protect yourself by avoiding exposure to the sun, especially midday sun, and wearing protective clothing. Everyone, regardless of risk, should avoid using tanning parlors.

Many doctors believe that the use of sunscreen should be a daily routine for people of all ages. Sunscreen should not, however, be regarded as the ultimate barrier against skin cancer. Even when you use sunscreen, you should still avoid prolonged exposure to the sun. When buying sunscreen, look for those that have any of the following ingredients, which help block both ultraviolet A and B (UVA and UVB) rays: benzophenones, oxybenzone, sulisobenzone, titanium dioxide, zinc oxide, and butyl methoxydibenzoylmethane, also known as avobenzone. Use a brand that has at least a sun protection factor (SPF) of 15 or higher. Apply sunscreen even on cloudy days, since 80 percent of the sun's harmful rays still reach your skin.

HEREDITY

Most cancers are related to lifestyle—diet, use of alcohol and tobacco, exercise—and environmental factors. Yet heredity is known to play a part in cancer risk. Here's some of what the experts know thus far.

Hereditary Cancer Patterns

Researchers have identified more than two hundred hereditary cancer patterns that can predispose people to certain cancers. This does not mean that everyone who has a particular cancer or disease history will get the same condition but instead that there is an increased risk for the disease. For example:

- People with a family history of prostate, lung, breast, colorectal, and gastric cancers have an increased risk of developing these same cancers.

- People with a family history of adenomatous polyps, Gardner's syndrome, hereditary nonpolyposis colorectal cancer, and familial adenomatous polyposis have an increased risk of developing colorectal cancer.

- Chances of developing ovarian cancer are higher in women with a family history of Lynch syndrome II, breast-ovarian cancer syndrome, and site-specific ovarian cancer syndrome.

- A personal history of diabetes, estrogen replacement therapy, high blood pressure, colorectal cancer, breast cancer, and no children increases a woman's chances of getting ovarian cancer.

- People with a personal history of chronic obstructive pulmonary disease, emphysema, chronic bronchitis, Hodgkin's disease, or lung scarring have an increased risk of lung cancer.

These are just a few of the possible factors that can increase a person's risk of getting cancer. Much still depends on your lifestyle and your exposure to environmental factors. Consult with your physician about these and other conditions to see if you are a candidate for preventive screening for cancer.

Evaluating Cancer Risk and Cancer Screening

For people with a personal or family history that suggests a possible increased risk of cancer, cancer screening is advisable, and genetic counseling and/or testing is an option. There are some cancer-screening tests, however, that are recommended for everyone based on sex and/or age. These screening tests, along with some others, are explained briefly below. Consult with your physician if you have any questions about any of these procedures, or contact the American Cancer Society for information on how to do self-examinations.

• *Breast Self-Examination.* All women should perform this simple examination every month. Premenopausal women should do it during the week following their menstrual period; postmenopausal women should choose one easy-to-remember day, such as the first or last day each month. Any change in breast size, color, skin texture, tenderness, or nipple retraction should be reported to your physician.

• *Skin Self-Examination.* Three to four times a year, everyone should examine all areas of their skin, including underarms, back, buttocks, and between the toes. A hand-held mirror can be used to check hard-to-see spots, or a partner or spouse can help.

• *Testicular Self-Examination.* To check for testicular cancer, men should examine their testicles for hard masses several times a year. This examination is best done after a warm shower or bath.

• *Stool Blood Test*. This test detects possible colorectal cancer. Fecal samples collected three days in a row are examined for blood. Recommended yearly after age fifty.

• *Sputum Cytology*. Sputum samples from three consecutive days are collected and examined for evidence of lung cancer or a precancerous condition.

• *Pelvic Exam*. Performed by a physician for early detection of cervical cancer, it is recommended that women have this examination once a year beginning at age eighteen or when they become sexually active, whichever comes first.

• *Prostate-Specific Antigen Test*. A blood test used to screen for prostate cancer.

• *Digital Rectal Exam*. The physician inserts a lubricated, gloved finger into the rectum to detect any abnormalities that may signal cancer of the colon, rectum, or prostate. This screening is recommended yearly for all adults older than forty.

• *Pap Test*. A screening tool for cervical cancer in which cell samples are scraped from the cervix and upper vagina and then analyzed. It is recommended that women have this test once a year beginning at age eighteen or when they become sexually active, whichever comes first.

• *Mammography*. A mammogram is an X ray of the breast used for early detection of breast tumors. Yearly mammograms are recommended for women older than fifty. Doctors still disagree on the need for mammograms for women between forty and fifty. Follow your physician's advice.

• *Sigmoidoscopy*. Use of a flexible, lighted instrument called an endoscope to view the esophagus and stomach. Recommended every three to five years for people fifty and older.

• *Colonoscopy*. A screening and diagnostic test that utilizes a lighted, flexible instrument called a colonoscope to view the colon.

Positive findings on any of the above screening procedures may lead to further testing by your physician.

Genetic Counseling and Screening

Genetic counseling and genetic screening are not routine procedures in the U.S., but they are available and recommended for individuals who have concerns and/or meet the basic criteria of hereditary cancer. Those criteria apply to families that have:

- Members who have cancer that developed fifteen to twenty years earlier than normal
- Members in which cancer has affected more than one close relative
- Close relatives (parents or siblings) who have more than one form of cancer
- Cancer that affects more than one generation

People who seek genetic counseling and screening include those who are contemplating pregnancy, women who are considering hormone replacement therapy, and those who have unresolved fears about their chances of developing certain cancers so they can take appropriate measures to lessen their risk. Become familiar with the warning signs of the particular type of cancer about which you are concerned. Organizations that can help you investigate patterns of hereditary cancer in your family are listed in Appendix A.

OBESITY

Although not conclusive, many experts believe obesity increases the risk for some cancers. Among women the risk for breast cancer is especially significant after menopause, because the excess body fat produces extra estrogen, which in turn triggers abnormal cell growth. Among women who are severely obese (40 percent or more above ideal weight), the risk for uterine cancer and ovarian cancer increases.

The risk of colorectal cancer also increases for those who are obese. According to a study in the *Journal of the National Cancer Institute*, "The principal sites of excess cancer mortality among overweight men (but not women) were found to be in the colon and the rectum."

A healthful, cancer-preventive diet as outlined in Chapters 4 and 7, along with a regular exercise program that includes thirty minutes of moderate activity at least five days a week, can help men and women lose excess weight. If you are obese and want to lose weight, consult with your physician or health-care practitioner to set up an appropriate nutrition and exercise plan.

ENVIRONMENTAL FACTORS

It is estimated that environmental exposures to toxic substances account for about 5 percent of all cancer deaths (this does not include contamination of food; see Chapter 5 for information about pesticides in food). Although this figure may seem insignificant, it also may be erroneous, as scientists are discovering more and more each day about the effects of synthetic and natural compounds on health and how they may trigger cancer and other medical conditions.

Another statistic of interest is that approximately 15 percent of lung cancer is linked to prolonged exposure to carcinogens in the environment, both in the home and the workplace. The three most important factors—secondhand smoke, asbestos, and radon—are responsible for an estimated five thousand deaths per year.

Below I look at some of the known and possible carcinogens in the environment and how you can avoid them or lessen their effect on your health.

Asbestos

Until the late 1970s, a fibrous material called asbestos was used extensively as insulation and in fireproofing, shingles, siding, floor and ceiling tiles, and in many appliances. That's when the U.S. Consumer Product Safety Commission banned its use. Asbestos can still be found in many homes and commercial buildings that were built or remodeled before the late 1970s.

Asbestos is a problem only if it is damaged or tampered with, which allows the fibers to become airborne. That's when they can be inhaled and lodged in lung tissue, where they cannot be removed. Asbestos has been linked to lung cancer and cancer of the larynx. Those at greatest risk are people who work with asbestos or who are exposed to it, and smokers. If you know or suspect that you have asbestos in your home or office, do not touch it. Call your state asbestos office and ask for the names of certified asbestos contractors. Even if the asbestos in your home is still intact, you may want to have it removed, enclosed, or encapsulated to eliminate or reduce the risk of contamination.

Radon

The Environmental Protection Agency estimates that up to twenty thousand cancer deaths a year can be attributed to radon. It is the second leading cause of lung cancer in the United States. This radioactive gas, which is produced by the natural breakdown of uranium in the earth, is believed to affect one in fifteen homes in America. These homes are built over bedrock that contains radium. The gas can enter the house through cracks in the foundation or floor, gaps in service pipes, construction joints, or cracks in the walls.

How do you know if radon is in your house? Radon is invisible, tasteless, and odorless. When it comes out of the earth and enters the atmosphere, it is virtually harmless. It is only when it dissipates into an enclosed area, such as a home, and becomes trapped that it accumulates and becomes deadly. You can test for radon with a radon test kit, available at most hardware stores and home centers. When buying a radon test kit, make sure the package says "Meets EPA Requirements." There are two types of home detection kits, both inexpensive and easy to use. The charcoal canister kit stays in the home for three to seven days before being mailed in for evaluation. Alpha-track detectors remain in the house for two to four weeks or longer before being sent in for analysis. A professional can come in and install monitoring devices that take readings over a period of time.

You can protect yourself against radon contamination by allowing lots of natural ventilation in your home. This is most important in the lowest level of your house, where the radon usually enters. Leaving windows open much of the time is not practical or safe for many people, however. A method of forced ventilation that draws outside air into the house or a heat recovery ventilator can be used as an alternative. Consult with a radon specialist to determine what is best for your home. Each state has a radon contact office. Look in the state government section of your telephone directory for the one in your state.

Secondhand Smoke

Secondhand smoke is defined as a combination of smoke from the burning end of a cigarette and the exhaled smoke of a smoker. In 1992, the EPA classified secondhand smoke as a Group A carcinogen. Items in Group A are the most dangerous cancer-causing agents.

About three thousand people a year die of lung cancer caused by secondhand smoke. If you do not smoke but live with someone who does, your chances of getting lung cancer increase by 30 percent. Secondhand smoke is also responsible for an alarming number of medical problems among children. According to Action on Smoking and Health, a nonprofit nonsmokers' rights organization, each year secondhand smoke is responsible for one million asthma attacks, 26,000 new cases of asthma, 300,000 cases of lower respiratory infection, and 1,000 infant deaths from sudden infant death syndrome.

Here are some things you can do to avoid secondhand smoke:

- In your home, ask family members to smoke outside or in just one room of the house. They may also smoke next to an open window. Better, urge them to quit.

- Ask guests not to smoke in your home.

- Patronize restaurants that are smoke-free.

- If smoking is allowed in your workplace (this is becoming much less common), make sure there are fair company policies for nonsmokers.

- Use fans and open windows when in an environment with smokers that you cannot change.

- Politely let smokers know that you'd appreciate if they did not smoke around you.

Pesticides in the Home and Garden

Pesticides are used by approximately seventy million households in the United States. And the selection of killers is wide. According to the National Home and Garden Pesticide Use Survey (1990) conducted by the EPA, there are more than 20,000 different household pesticide products containing more than 300 active ingredients and 1,700 inert ingredients. Disinfectants to kill fungus, viruses, and bacteria are the most used of pesticides in the home. Many disinfectants contain formaldehyde, which was classified as a possible human carcinogen in 1992.

To reduce your exposure to pesticides, use only products that are nontoxic. Use simple, antibacterial soaps and bleach for cleaning. For insect control, use biological controls (see Appendix A). Seal any crevices and cracks around windows and doors where insects can get into the house. Replace any screens that have holes and cracks where insects can get in. If you must use a pesticide, follow the safety directions on the product.

The use of pesticides specifically on the lawn and in the garden is rampant in the United States. According to a 1990 report from the National Academy of Sciences, American homeowners use five to ten pounds of pesticides per acre of lawn each year. This is ten times more pesticides than farmers use on their crops. Twelve of the most commonly used lawn pesticides are suspected carcinogens, and the EPA has a list of fifty-three pesticides that have been banned or severely restricted. (See list of severely restricted pesticides below.) These agents can very easily get into your home, groundwater, and garden vegetables, and they even affect your pets. Some of these contaminants, such as DDT, methoxychlor, toxaphene, dieldrin, endosulfan, chlordane, and aldrin, can reside in fatty tissue in the body, especially in the breast, and mimic estrogen. If the link between increased levels of estrogen and the risk of breast cancer is true, then these pesticides carry a significant cancer risk.

The dangers of pesticide use on lawns and gardens can be avoided by using biological controls. This includes the use of beneficial insects and naturally occurring bacteria. Contact your local county agricultural extension service for information.

SEVERELY RESTRICTED PESTICIDES

These pesticides are to be used by certified pesticide control applicators only. If you have pesticides that contain any of these chemicals, discard them at a hazardous-waste facility.

Arsenic trioxide	Heptachlor
Carbonfuran	Mercuric chloride
Chlordane	Mercurous chloride
Daminozide	Phenylmercury acetate
EDB	Tributyltin compounds

Chemicals in the Environment

More than seventy thousand chemicals are being used in some capacity in the United States. According to the U.S. Department of Labor Occupational Safety and Health Administration (OSHA), up to 160 of these chemicals could be proven carcinogens, and about 2,000 more could be potential cancer-causing agents. Many of these are found in industry, yet a good number are in your home and even in your medicine. Although there is a list of known carcinogens (discussed below), there is a much longer list of suspected carcinogens that have not been tested properly. In fact, only 10 percent of new chemicals have been adequately tested for their cancer-causing potential. And of the 120 substances identified as carcinogens during animal tests over the last twenty years, less than 10 percent have undergone epidemiological study by the National Cancer Institute or by industry.

A list of some of the known carcinogens that are still being used in the United States is given below. Remember that the list of suspected or possible carcinogens is reported to be in the tens of thousands by some experts.

• *Arsenic and arsenic compounds*. Although no longer manufactured in the United States, these compounds are still imported. Arsenic is found in pesticides and herbicides and may contaminate food and drinking water; it is associated with cancers of the lung, skin, and liver.

• *Asbestos*. Asbestos is no longer made in the United States, but many buildings still contain it and thus pose a danger. (See pages 147–148.)

• *Azathioprine*. A synthetic chemical administered to some patients with autoimmune diseases and patients with organ transplants. Azathioprine can cause non-Hodgkin's lymphoma and tumors in various organs.

• *Benzene*. Chemical used during the manufacture of paint, plastic, and adhesives. Perhaps the largest human exposure comes from gasoline, as benzene is a gasoline additive and is emitted into the atmosphere in automobile and bus exhaust. Benzene is linked with causing the cell mutation process that develops into leukemia.

• *Bis-chloromethyl ether*. Used in the manufacture of plastics. It is associated with lung cancer.

• *14-butanediol dimethanesulfonate*. This drug is used to treat leukemia, yet studies show that it may lead to the development of the same disease.

• *Chlorambucil*. A drug used to treat various forms of cancer. It may lead to the development of leukemia.

• *Chromium and chromium compounds*. These chemicals are used extensively in the textile and tanning industries, as protective coating for cars, and in paint, food, and industrial water treatment. Exposure has been linked with an increased risk of lung and other cancers.

• *Cyclophosphamide*. This anticancer drug is used to treat malignant melanoma, leukemia, lymphoma, and various other cancers, yet it can increase the risk for leukemia, bladder cancer, and other cancers.

• *Melphalan*. An anticancer drug used to treat ovarian and breast cancers and myeloma. Its use increases the risk of developing second primary cancers, especially leukemia.

• *Vinyl chloride*. This substance is used widely throughout industry because it is flame-retardant and cost-effective. It is a potent carcinogen that has been linked with lymphoma and cancers of the lung, liver, and brain among people who work with it.

Your only defense against these and other dangerous chemicals is education. Find out about possible toxic dumps in your area; learn about any chemicals that are used in your workplace; investigate the pollutants emitted by industries close to you.

OTHER CANCER RISKS

Some other cancer risks that don't fall into any of the above categories are reviewed here briefly.

Oral Contraceptives

Since the mid-1980s, there have been many studies of a possible increased risk of breast cancer among women who use oral contraceptives (the Pill). Evidence of a link has been mounting, yet a definitive answer is not possible. One reason is that there have been and continue to be many different versions of the Pill, which makes comparison studies impossible. On a positive note is the fact that the amount of estrogen and progesterone in the Pill is now much lower than it was when oral contraceptives were first formulated and the studies were initially done. Women are still awaiting a definitive answer however, regarding the possible cancer link.

Exercise

It is not exercise itself, but the lack of exercise that is a problem. What has exercise to do with cancer? Studies show that a healthy immune system is instrumental in preventing cancer, and regular exercise helps keep the immune system in optimal shape. Here are a few facts:

- Moderate exercise increases the amount of natural killer cells that circulate throughout the body. These cells are responsible for destroying tumor cells.
- Harvard University studies show a 25 to 50 percent lower incidence of colon cancer among people who exercise moderately.
- The risk of breast, ovarian, and uterine cancers is lower among women who exercise regularly. That's because exercise helps stabilize the estrogen level in the

body, and an abundance of estrogen is associated with abnormal cell growth and tumors in the female reproductive organs.

• Although not yet conclusive, studies suggest that exercise helps reduce the risk of prostate cancer in men by lowering testosterone levels.

How much exercise is enough? In 1993, the American College of Sports Medicine, the Centers for Disease Control, and several other health organizations defined it as thirty minutes or more of moderate exercise (a brisk walk or low-impact aerobics, for example) at least five times a week. Incorporate physical activity into your daily routine when you can: Take the stairs instead of the elevator, or take a brisk walk during lunch or a coffee break, for example.

Sex

Women have a progressively increased risk of developing cervical cancer as the number of their sexual partners increases. Their risk also is greater as the number of sexual partners their partner(s) have had increases. Of much greater concern regarding multiple sexual partners is the risk of AIDS.

A LAST WORD

You can improve your health and the health of your family when you add the power of some very fragile but potent sprouts to your diet. As little as 1 ounce a week can reduce your risk of getting cancer by 50 percent. When combined with other cancer- and disease-preventive foods and positive lifestyle habits, broccoli sprouts can be an insurance policy for wellness. Make them a regular part of your menu plans and experiment with new ways to incorporate them into your diet. *Bon appetit* and good health!

Appendix A

ORGANIZATIONS AND PRODUCT SOURCES

Cancer and Cancer-Prevention Information

Alcoholics Anonymous
475 Riverside Drive
New York, NY 10115
212-870-3400

American Cancer Society
1599 Clifton Road, NE
Atlanta, GA 30329
404-320-3333; 800-ACS-2345

American Lung Association—Freedom from Smoking
1740 Broadway
New York, NY 10019
212-315-8700

Center for Substance Abuse Treatment Referral Hotline
11426 Rockville Pike
Suite 410
Rockville, MD 20852
800-662-HELP

"Food, Nutrition, and the Prevention of Cancer: A Global
   Perspective."
For a free brochure about the report, call 800-843-8114, ext. 723, and
ask for the FNS publication.

Hereditary Cancer Institute
Creighton University
Department of Preventive Medicine
2500 California Plaza
Omaha, NE 68178

National Cancer Institute
Office of Cancer Communications
Bldg. 31, Room 10A24
Bethesda, MD 20892
800-4-CANCER
Call for booklets about specific cancer types and other cancer-related topics, such as "Clearing the Air: How to Quit Smoking . . . and Quit for Keeps." Also provides referrals to genetic-counseling departments in your area.

U.S. Environmental Protection Agency
Information Access Branch
Public Information Center
401 M Street, SW
Washington, DC 20460
202-260-2080
Information and booklets, such as "A Citizen's Guide to Radon."

Environmental and Pesticide Issues

Assistance Information Service (EPA) Asbestos Hotline
401 M Street, SW
Washington, DC 20460
202-554-1404

Mothers for Natural Law
515-472-2809
Information about genetically engineered foods

National Coalition Against the Misuse of Pesticides
701 E Street SE
Suite 200
Washington, DC 20003
202-543-5450
Information on the health effects of and alternatives to pesticides

National Coalition for Alternatives to Pesticides
PO Box 1393
Eugene, OR 97440
503-344-5044
Information on nontoxic ways to eliminate hazards introduced by fungi and pests

Natural Food Associates
PO Box 210
Atlanta, TX 75551
800-594-2136
Information on organic growing, pesticide use, and human health

Rachel Carson Council
8940 Jones Mill Road
Chevy Chase, MD 20815
301-652-1877
Offers free publications and assistance to people who have problems
with pesticides

Health Practitioners

American Society of Clinical Hypnosis
2200 East Devon Avenue
Suite 291
Des Plaines, IL 60018
708-297-3317

National Commission for the Certification of Acupuncturists
1424 16th Street, NW
Suite 501
Washington, DC 20036
202-232-1404

Society for Clinical and Experimental Hypnosis
6728 Old McLean Village Drive
McLean, VA 22101
703-556-9222

Food and Nutrition Information

American Academy of Orthomolecular Medicine
900 North Federal Highway
Boca Raton, FL 33432
800-847-3802

American Botanical Council
PO Box 201660
Austin, TX 78720
800-373-7105

Center for Science in the Public Interest
1875 Connecticut Avenue, NW
Suite 300
Washington, DC 20009
202-332-9111
Publishers of *The Nutrition Action Health Letter*

Herb Research Foundation
1007 Pearl Street
Suite 200
Boulder CO 80302
303-449-2265

North American Vegetarian Society
PO Box 72
Dolgeville, NY 13329
518-568-7970

Physicians Committee for Responsible Medicine
PO Box 6322
Washington, DC 20015
202-686-2210

Preventive Medicine Research Institute
Dean Ornish, MD
900 Bridgeway
Suite 2
Sausalito, CA 94965
415-332-2525

Soy Protein Council
1255 23rd Street, NW
Suite 850
Washington, DC 20037
202-467-6610

United Soybean Hotline
800-TALK SOY
Recipes and information about soy and soy products

Vegetarian Education Network
PO Box 3347
West Chester, PA 19380
215-696-VNET

Vegetarian Resource Group
PO Box 1463
Baltimore, MD 21203
410-366-8343

Organic and Plant-Based Food Manufacturers

Arrowhead Mills
PO Box 2059
Hereford, TX 79045
806-364-0730
Organic grains and flours

Eden Foods
701 Tecumseh Road
Clinton, MI 49236
517-456-7424
Edensoy: organic soy beverages

Ivy Foods
7613 South Prospector Drive
Salt Lake City, UT 84121
801-943-7664
Wheat-based "meat" products

Morningstar Farms
Worthington Foods
Worthington, OH 43085
614-885-9511
Meatless products: breakfast links, breakfast patties, deli franks, and others

Nasoya
23 Jytek Dr.
Leominster MA 01453
800-229-8638
Tofu, Nayonaisse

Purity Foods
2871 W. Jolly Road
Okemos, MI 48864
800-99-SPELT
Pastas

Soyco Foods
2441 Viscount Row
Orlando, FL 32809
407-855-6600
Cheese alternatives

Westbrae
1065 E. Walnut Street
Carson, CA 90746
800-769-6455
Soy beverages

White Wave
1990 N. 57th Court
Boulder, CO 80301
303-443-3470
Meatless chicken products

Appendix B

SUGGESTED READING AND SOURCES

Altman, Roberta. *Every Woman's Handbook for Preventing Cancer*. New York: Pocket Books, 1996.

Balch, James, M.D., and Phyllis A. Balch. *Prescription for Nutritional Healing*. Garden City Park, NY: Avery Publishing, 1990.

Barnard, Neal, M.D. *The Power of Your Plate: A Plan for Better Living*. Summertown, TN: Book Publishing Company, 1995.

Baron-Faust, Rita. *Breast Cancer: What Every Woman Should Know*. New York: Hearst Books, 1995.

The Basic Formula to Create Community Supported Agriculture. Indian Line Farm, RR 3, Box 85, Great Barrington, MA 01230 ($10).

Braunstein, Mark Matthew. *The Sprout Garden: The Indoor Growers' Guide to Gourmet Sprouts*. Summertown, TN: Book Publishing Company, 1993.

Brody, Jane E. *The New York Times Book of Health*. New York: Random House, 1997.

Cassileth, Barrie R., Ph.D. *The Alternative Medicine Handbook*. New York: Norton, 1998.

Cooper, Kenneth H., M.D. *Advanced Nutritional Therapies*. Nashville: Thomas Nelson, 1996.

———. *Dr. Kenneth H. Cooper's Antioxidant Revolution*. Nashville: Thomas Nelson, 1995.

Fahey, Jed W. "Broccoli Sprouts: An Exceptionally Rich Source of Inducers of Enzymes that Protect against Chemical Carcinogens." *Proc Natl Acd Sci* 94 (1997): 10367–72.

Fox, Barry. *Foods to Heal By*. New York: St. Martin's Press, 1996.

Fox, Nicols. *Spoiled: The Dangerous Truth about a Food Chain Gone Haywire*. New York: Basic Books, 1997.

Green, Nancy Sokol. *Poisoning Our Children*. Chicago: Noble Press, 1991.

Haas, Robert, M.S. *Permanent Remissions*. New York: Simon & Schuster, 1997.

Harte, John, et al. *Toxics A to Z: A Guide to Everyday Pollution Hazards*. Berkeley: University of California Press, 1991.

Hobbs, Christopher. *Medicinal Mushrooms*. Capitola, CA: Botanica Press, 1986.

Holt, Tamara. *Bean Power*. New York: Bantam Doubleday Dell, 1993.

Jones, Helen Taylor. *Grain Power*. New York: Bantam Doubleday Dell, 1993.

Keane, Maureen, M.S., and Daniella Chace, M.S. *What to Eat if You Have Cancer*. Chicago: Contemporary Books, 1996.

Klaper, Michael, M.D. *Vegan Nutrition Pure and Simple*. Maui, HI: Gentle World, 1987.

Kradjian, Robert M., M.D. *Save Yourself from Breast Cancer*. New York: Berkley Publishing Group, 1994.

Krause, Carol. *How Healthy Is Your Family Tree?* New York: Macmillan, 1994.

Kushi, Michio. *The Macrobiotic Approach to Cancer*. Garden City Park, NY: Avery Publishing, 1991.

Lappé, Frances M. *Diet for a Small Planet*. Rev. ed. New York: Ballantine Books, 1975.

Larimore, Bertha B. *Sprouting For All Seasons: How and What to Sprout Including Delicious, Easy to Prepare Recipes*. Bountiful, VT: Horizon Publishing, 1997.

Levenstein, Mary Kerney. *Everyday Cancer Risks and How to Avoid Them*. Garden City Park, NY: Avery Publishing, 1992.

Messina, Mark, and Virginia Messina. *The Simple Soybean and Your Health*. Garden City Park, NY: Avery Publishing, 1994.

Moss, Ralph W., Ph.D. *Cancer Therapy: The Independent Consumers' Guide to Nontoxic Treatment and Prevention*. New York: Equinox Press, 1992.

Murray, Michael T., N.D. *The Healing Power of Herbs*. 2d ed. Rocklin, CA: Prima Publishing, 1995.

Reuben, Carolyn. *Antioxidants: Your Complete Guide*. Rocklin, CA: Prima Publishing, 1995.

Robbins, John. *Diet for a New America: How Your Food Choices Affect Your Health, Happiness, and the Future of Life on Earth*. Walpole, NH: Stillpoint Publishing, 1987.

———. *May All Be Fed*. New York: Morrow, 1992.

Sellmann, Per. *The Complete Sprouting Book*. Wellingborough, Northamptonshire, England: Turnstone Press, 1981.

Sharma, Hari, M.D. *Freedom From Disease: How to Control Free Radicals*. Toronto: Veda Publishing, 1993.

Taylor, Nadine, M.S. *Green Tea: The Natural Secret for a Healthier Life*. New York: Kensington Publishing, 1998.

Wasserman, Debbie. *Simply Vegan: Quick Vegetarian Meals*. Baltimore: Vegetarian Resource Group, 1991.

Weil, Andrew, M.D. *Natural Health, Natural Medicine: 8 Weeks to Optimum Health*. Boston: Houghton Mifflin, 1990.

Werbach, Melvyn, M.D. *Healing Through Nutrition*. New York: HarperCollins, 1993.

———. *Nutritional Influences on Illness*. 2d ed. Tarzana, CA: Third Line Press, 1993.

Wigmore, Ann. *The Sprouting Book*. Garden City Park, NY: Avery Publishing, 1986.

Winawer, Sidney J., M.D., and Moshe Shike, M.D. *Cancer Free*. New York: Simon & Schuster, 1995.

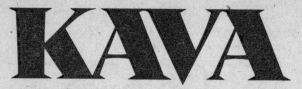